the
Hardgainer
Solution

The Training and Diet Plans for Building a
Better Body, Gaining Muscle, and
Overcoming Your Genetics

SCOTT ABEL

edited by Perry Mykleby

Published by:

Scott Abel

© Copyright Scott Abel

ISBN-13: 978-1511703598
ISBN-10: 1511703598

TABLE *of* CONTENTS

Part 3.
The Hardgainer's Diet Solution

Part 4.
The Complete List of Workouts & Diet Plans

ABOUT *the* **AUTHOR**

Scott Abel has been involved in the diet, fitness, and bodybuilding industries for over four decades. He has written for, or been featured in magazines like Muscle & Fitness, Flex, Muscle Mag, T-Nation, and many more.

The Hardgainer Solution is based on more than just Scott's knowledge of exercise physiology and workout program design; it has also been tested and tweaked based on Scott's experiences working with hundreds of clients for over thirty years.

Part 1.

The Truth About Hardgainers
and the Logic Behind This
Program

The Hardgainer Dilemma

I've spent the last couple of years reviewing my notes and coming up with new strategies to help one of the toughest demographics out there – the Hardgainers – and I'm really on to something with what I've come up with, and I'm excited to get it out there.

Most Hardgainers already know they're Hardgainers.

If this is you, no one needs to tell you that you are Hardgainer: you've tried every workout program out there and you still feel frustrated by a lack of results. Your results simply don't reflect your efforts. I get it.

But some of you may be Hardgainers and not even realize it. This means you could be making more progress than you have so far – if you start following the right protocol in the right way.

Being a Hardgainer is not just limited to being a skinny ectomorph. That's easy to categorize, but it's not the whole story.

Here are the other common signs that someone is a Hardgainer:

- Training for years and not changing your body shape.

- Training for years and not gaining heavier body weight from yearly muscle mass increases.

- Training for years and people still ask you if you work out.

- Training for years and no muscle maturity and development shows on you with your shirt off.

However, there are other aspects to being a Hardgainer.

For example, you lose muscle as you age. This is true even if you work out, and even if you've got pretty good genetics.

I watch pro sports like NFL football, and at certain positions they say that a player is "getting old" when barely into his 30s.

Well, developing a physique becomes more challenging as you age as well. Research shows that men in their 50s are a new category of consumers in cosmetic surgery and body transformation interest.

There is a natural slow loss of muscle that begins around age 35, whether you work out or not. Even myself, I was able to maintain a fairly high level of muscle mass till I turned 50.

After age 50, I would now also consider myself a Hardgainer, because I know and understand the ongoing muscle and performance loss that accompanies aging. The benefit I have is "know-how" and people still comment on my physique, even at this age.

But make no mistake, I've had a personal interest in addressing the Hardgainer issue and I'm really on to something with this program.

And to reiterate: someone older – say someone in his 40s – who is just starting to work out to transform his physique… this person is a Hardgainer from the get-go.

However, properly addressing the Hardgainer issue required me looking at this differently. First of all, every Hardgainer is unique metabolically.

That is something no one ever talks about.

But it's true.

Moreover someone tall and lanky is likely to be a Hardgainer because the lever systems of long arms and legs put their physiques at a disadvantage when trying to overload muscles. Long limbs mean having to move resistance through a greater range of motion, often with less support from stabilizing and guiding muscles.

So someone who is taller and older for instance, is really likely to be a Hardgainer.

This also means that a tall and lanky person is less likely to be able to lift "heavier" weights: and "heavier weights" have always been the "myth" of the solution to the Hardgainer issue! Not any more!

I developed Metabolic Enhancement Training (or "MET training") beginning back around 2004, and since then I've had a decade or more to observe the feedback of my coaching clients, and the people who've purchased my MET programs. I was also able to cross-reference this with feedback from my clients who used my Innervation Training methodology protocols (the more traditional "body part" programs for building muscle).

I realized that for Hardgainers, industry experts (including myself!) tended to address the issue too myopically. When you look at the comments and programs aimed at Hardgainers, the discussion is always about training for the Hardgainer, but only in a very specific sense.

There are other elements of training that don't get enough consideration.

First is recovery. I started to address the elements of recovery, both within workouts, and between workouts. If Hardgainers are unique metabolically, then intra-workout recovery and inter-workout recovery are serious matters of consideration. Training affects their recovery, and their recovery affects their training.

No one was properly addressing this, at least not without sacrificing the volume and intensity needed for growth.

And along with these, the intensity factor is another consideration for the Hardgainer – a consideration that to my mind has until now been misconstrued.

Many experts insinuate that Hardgainers just don't train intensely enough. That may be true for some, but you just can't paint the whole demographic of the Hardgainer with that same brush.

I've also experienced the opposite. In my heyday, everyone wanted to work out with me, *and some of my best training partners I would call "Hardgainers."* They could hang with me rep for rep, where other plate-heads who had much more muscle just couldn't – yet they didn't have the physique development to show for it. Why? This wasn't being addressed by the industry!

I've come to learn and embrace that it's because these weren't the right workouts for their unique metabolic needs.

Many of the workout programs that Hardgainers follow are simply unsuited to their genetic situation. One question I would ask of any Hardgainer: if you *are* a true Hardgainer, why are you going to hardcore bodybuilders for workout guidance?

These guys are genetically suited for developing muscle, or they wouldn't be competing to begin with.

Then you add in the use of a myriad of performance enhancing drugs and the question begs, how is following what they do addressing what YOU actually need as a Hardgainer?

In terms of intensity, for the Hardgainer's unique metabolic profile, the Hardgainer may actually be training "too hard." That's right: that is what I just said!

It may not sound "macho" enough for the "blood, sweat and tears" attitude of the modern training world, but it is indeed part of what is holding the Hardgainer back.

And so is this emphasis on body part workout days (one day per body part). In terms of intra-workout recovery and inter-workout recovery I've discovered that this approach is NOT well-suited to the Hardgainer.

I'm really onto something with my Hardgainer's Solution, which covers not just a whole year of training, but also covers how to approach the Hardgainer's nutritional needs as well.

My coaching clients exposed to this new approach report making great gains... FINALLY.

But it requires a new direction in thinking. The Hardgainer is easily over-trained. The solution is to be under-trained – not by training less often (because muscles still demand constant stimulation in order to grow), but by looking at your training differently.

This is what I am hoping *The Hardgainer Solution* offers. I'm extremely excited about this project!

Why the Hardgainer Solution Will Work For You

If you're a Hardgainer and you think you've tried everything...

...then, frankly, you probably haven't.

The reason I say this is because while all these other programs aimed at Hardgainers may differ in degree, they don't differ in design.

These are programs that are usually all "load-based" programs. They are programs founded upon lifting "more weight," but if this were truly the solution to the Hardgainer dilemma, then you would already be there in terms of desired results, wouldn't you?

These programs may even be "good and reasonable" programs. The problem is they come from the perspective of program design, and NOT from the perspective of the Hardgainer dilemma.

The *Hardgainer's Solution* is different because it is a reps-based program. The reps are the point of emphasis – and high reps at that. Exercise selection and how much you lift are not the emphasis.

So, instead of the program being founded upon "lifting more weight," my *Hardgainer's Solution* is founded upon the notion of lifting weight better.

I have been doing this program myself for close to two years now. (Yes, I've been on the same program for two years.)

A quick anecdote:

Every year I take an annual vacation in Aruba. Because I'm able to stay there a long time, I now work out while I'm there, mostly just to get out of the burning hot sun. While I was training in the hotel gym during my last trip, there were a few other people working out there as well.

One fellow was a thin man, about my age, and he looked like maybe he was a runner. I asked him if I could work in with him on a piece of equipment. He offered instead to "get out of my way" because I am going to have to change the weight compared to what he was lifting.

He was insinuating that because of the appearance of my physique, he assumed I would be changing the weights on the machine to lift much heavier than what he was lifting.

And I did indeed have to change the weight when working in with him. But you should have seen the look on his face when I made the weight "lighter" than what he was lifting.

But this is the nature of the *Hardgainer Solution Workouts.*

They are higher reps-based protocols and not load-based protocols. This takes a page out of my Innervation Training Methodology that dictates that for most people it is a myth that if "you train for strength, development will come."

How often have you heard that one? But it's simply not true. For instance my colleague Kevin Weiss, World Champion Powerlifter, has coached many male and female powerlifters who can lift more weight than I can in terms of "strength." Yet they don't show near the level of development I do. You do the math.

Furthermore, as research in my book *The Abel Approach* points out, training for muscular strength is not connected to achieving muscle development. This quote by David Behm is used in *The Abel Approach*:

"Maximum strength training methods, with their high intensity of resistance, but low volume of work, do NOT elicit substantial muscle hypertrophy. Therefore, a higher volume of work – greater than 6 reps and with multiple sets – these are both needed to ensure a critical concentration of intracellular amino acids to stimulate protein synthesis."

The Hardgainers solution gets back to the reality to train for development... PERIOD. Make that the priority.

You do this by realizing that the weights don't work the muscles; it's the muscles that work the weights.

This is a very important distinction regarding "intention" when it comes to working out. That fellow I worked in with in the gym in Aruba couldn't believe

I was training with lighter weights than he was – given I have advanced muscle development and he had very, very little.

But what the Hardgainer Solution workouts do is go beyond the "greater than six reps and with multiple sets" quote that I just used above. You see the Hardgainer Solution does indeed cover "the greater than 6 reps with multiple sets" prescription set out above – but so did all my previous Innervation Training programs. So by itself there was nothing new there.

What is "new," and what I've finally figured out, is how to amalgamate this formula to the rest and recovery needs of the true Hardgainer.

And this is why and how The Hardgainer Solution is superior to what I've seen out there so far. It goes the extra mile in considering the Hardgainer trainee demographic – not just from the perspective of the principles involved, but including the Hardgainer's unique metabolic need for recovery both within workouts and between workouts.

This is a very unique combination that finally targets the Hardgainer as a specific and unique training demographic.

Research has shown that angle of contraction can be just as important – or even more important for muscle recruitment – than the intensity of contraction. (See my book The Abel Approach for more references on this.)

The Hardgainer's Solution takes advantage of this by mixing up the order of the exercises, the order of the reps, and constantly varying the angles of contraction with different exercises.

This veers away totally from the usual "bench, squat, and deadlift" emphasis of most programs targeted at "gaining strength" in traditional lifts, which pretend to be a solution for the Hardgainer dilemma. (In fact I don't even use deadlifts at all in my Hardgainer solutions workouts, for reasons explained in the breakdown of the program).

A final anecdote:

Just the other day I was walking through the grocery store doing my grocery shopping.

An older couple behind me suddenly began talking to me: "How long have you been working out?" the man asked.

I replied, "Oh, I just try to exercise, I'm retired from that stuff."

"Naw, you wouldn't know that by looking at you," he said.

And he went on, talking my ear off regarding training and the like. It's obvious my Hardgainer solution workouts are working – even working on me, at my age.

Since I've been doing them, I've gotten comments like this all the time, and reactions like I got in the gym in Aruba as well.

What's that old saying from that hair restoration commercial? "I'm not only the owner, I'm a client."

The Hardgainer solution works, for Hardgainers and non-Hardgainers alike. But it's finally a program designed for the true Hardgainer. I'm excited to get it out to you.

One of My First "Tests" of the Hardgainer Solution

Once I had my "Eureka" moment and came up with the main ideas for the Hardgainer's Solution, I knew I had to test it out on myself and others.

Of course I had several clients who were great candidates for trying it out, and because they were clients, I was able to observe and tweak the HGS along the way.

One of my clients who fit the definition of "Hardgainer" is a young lad named Fausto Meloni, from Italy. Fausto is also a diabetic, so nutritional balance and training balance were a good test for the application of he HGS protocol.

Fausto Meloni
& the Hardgainer Application

At first, I assigned the whole body workouts to Fausto during his vacation in the summer of 2013.

He didn't have much equipment to work with, so I was able to assign a slightly stripped down "unplugged" version of the HGS protocol I was working on at the time.

I told him he could exercise up to seven time per week on this protocol, but that he was to keep intensity dialed back to about 60-70% Perceived Exertion. What happened next, surprised even me!

In the beginning, as a client, Fausto hated change. Any program change we did, he would report he didn't "like it," and then several weeks later he would "train into it," as I say, and all would be well.

But with the HGS workouts, he fell in love with this program right away (his words). He reported that he loved how invigorating the workouts felt, but without leaving him exhausted.

He definitely liked what I wrote into this program by design which is "stimulate don't annihilate" the muscles. And this was exactly what he was experiencing. Previous to this Fausto had been doing body part days, MET training, online hardcore training: the typical desperate route most Hardgainers take, pinballing from program to program without addressing that their specific needs are different as Hardgainers.

But this was finally a program aimed at his needs as a Hardgainer, and he was loving it from the get-go, something I'd never expected, but which makes total sense in retrospect.

The way the workouts are structured around body part training, by combining various body parts in whole body workouts with undulating rep schemes, was something his body responded to immediately.

For him, the missing ingredient was the use of a *variety* of ranges and planes of motion for stimulation, done in a way that didn't lead to burnout from going beyond "stimulation" such that the Hardgainer's body couldn't recover, within workouts and between workouts.

And this recovery element of the Hardgainer was something I'd explained before in other articles, but now I was witnessing the theory actually working beautifully in application and practice.

Even though the number of sets would mount over the course of the week, training body parts and parts of body parts within whole body complexes (e.g. separated heads of the delts on separate days) allowed for the kind of recovery so necessary for the Hardgainer.

And the more Fausto did these workouts, the more he liked them – the better he felt – and most importantly – the further he progressed, which was something he could see and feel.

Moreover, because of the reps emphasis of the program, he got further and further away from focusing on "how much" weight he used in a given exercise, and he started truly "feeling" the working muscles. This is a very advanced trainee experience, something many trainees never truly, fully understand.

But once again it's written into the program design because of the higher reps involved and the way the complexes are laid out.

Fausto reported finally being able to feel muscles that he never felt before in his workouts, something that was previously extremely frustrating for him. More importantly he was noticing his weaker body parts and the sides of his body catching up with everything else. In other words he was having a more "balanced" experience of his workouts. And of course this fed his motivation even more.

Previously Fausto was a lot like other Hardgainers I had witnessed over the years – he couldn't handle a lot of volume, yet as a Hardgainer more volume is exactly what is needed. As with all Hardgainers, it was a *Catch*-22.

The more volume he attempted in training, the less he recovered and the faster he burned out and hit a wall. But with the HGS workouts the body is taught to handle more volume day-to-day, week-to-week, which allows for recovery BECAUSE OF the way these workouts sessions are laid out. The basic elements of the HGS design is as follows:

1) Focusing on whole body workouts;

2) Focusing on undertraining in intensity;

3) Focusing more on rep variations, mostly higher reps, rather than focusing on loads used;

4) Having inter-workout and intra-workout recovery written into the program.

Now Fausto can handle 20-plus sets of training for a body part spread over a week, whereas before he could only "honeymoon" on that much volume and then burn out quickly with nothing to show for it.

I'm quite pleased with the results my clients are getting from the HGS workouts.

Here's Fausto's Account:

In summer of 2013 Coach Abel directed me to do a new program for the August month only, because I was on vacation and I didn't have that much equipment to work with. So for a single month he gave me a full body program that I could also do everyday, up to 7 sessions every week.

To my huge surprise this program was a real revelation to me, and I fell in love it with immediately.

At first I enjoyed how every day I felt I was training intensely, but without killing myself, and how I was looking forward to train again workout after workout.

Later I started to like how training with a single exercise per body part would make me focus on the hit zone tremendously and how at the end of each workout I felt that specific part stimulated enough and optimally to grow.

For example there were days where I would train my upper chest and felt my upper chest only, contracting and responding; or I could train delts and feel the central side of them, or their front/back side according to my workout and that day's exercise selection.

Over time I started to like it even more, because training each muscle daily even with few sets, my mind muscle connection improved in a way I wouldn't even think possible.

I started to feel each muscle contracting from the very first rep to the last, and I'd feel it on each muscle group, which was unexpected, because I'd always had trouble feeling my muscles overall – particularly my triceps and legs.

Workout after workout instead, not only have those particularly muscles started responding, but I can now feel exactly which muscle each exercise is hitting – the specific head of a given muscle, such as triceps or biceps, the outer part of my legs, the inner drop and so on.

Finally, after even more time on the program, I had one last surprise: not only had my muscles started to develop more fully ("filling" those "holes" I'd had), but even those asymmetric differences I had from one part to another started disappearing.

Now that I've switched to a different program I've truly noticed how the Hardgainer solution program increased my workload capacity and has allowed me to train with high volume in a way I just couldn't before.

I've always had a real hard time training with high volume because my body would just hit a wall. My muscles would start to get flat after a while, and not respond properly, so that I couldn't train with the intensity I wanted to.

Now it's just the opposite! My body responds extremely well to high volume training (I'm talking about 20+ sets for body part) and this is again a surprise which I've never experienced before.

What You've Been TOLD About Training

Before I get into explaining the nuts and bolts of the program and the diet strategy of this approach for Hardgainers, it's necessary to discuss a few important things, so that you get the most out of it.

If you are a Hardgainer, then chances are you've tried many, many different programs to develop your physique. You may have tried many different diets as well. But you don't build a body with a diet. You build a body with training and workouts. You build a body with proper, progressive, planned programming. Your diet complements your training.

I've looked over practically all the programs out there that promise the Hardgainer a better body.

Almost all of them are fundamentally flawed. Why? They are fundamentally flawed because they look at muscle development through the lens of old, worn-out traditional frames of thinking. Most of you have been told that you need to work to "get strong" and then that is how you build your body.

But this is only partially true, and it's completely misleading without proper context. There are many different kinds of strength, and not many of them lead to a better-developed physique. This is a big and long-standing myth in the bodybuilding and fitness industry.

You've been told to train for strength and development will come. But the real truth is that if you are a Hardgainer, you should train for development and strength will come.

Also note that the kind of strength I am talking about here is not one-rep max lift strength. That is known as "limit strength" and it is NOT the way to build and enhance a physique. The fact is, you can have a lousy one-rep max and have a huge, ripped physique. (I have never had great one-rep max numbers, and I only developed my physique once I stopped trying for big one-rep maxes.) And yes, you can have an amazing one-rep max and look like a couch potato.

Let's talk more about size versus strength, and about training for real development.

"Heavier is Better" is a Myth

Contrary to the one-rep max (1RM) strength theorists, it's not the weight that works the muscles; it's the muscles that work the weights. Read that over 10 times.

This is an important part of your biofeedback and the internal cues of training, which I will talk more about. It is also a departure from a focus on "how much" is on the bar lifted for how many reps.

This is an important switch in emphasis to internal aspects of performance, such as a perceived sense of exertion and affect, the actual angle of contraction of the muscle, muscle shortening, muscle activation potential, and so on.

It's an emphasis on how much stress a muscle is under; not how much weight is being lifted. This is the beginning of training maturity not measured in numbers, but felt in experience. The focus becomes, as I said, not on how much a trainee "can" lift, but rather on how much a trainee *should* lift for the desired effects.

How much you lift is not nearly as important as how hard (how intensely, how explosively) you lift. The "heavier is better" argument is a myth that prevents many of us from getting results in terms of physique enhancements.

J Atha, in 1981, concluded from a review of the academic research that, "from these studies, one begins to believe that the importance of load magnitude may have been exaggerated."

Let me give you two really clear examples from opposite ends of the spectrum:

I like to use Tom Platz and "Dr. Squat" Fred Hatfield as examples in my seminars.

Tom Platz had the first set of truly freaky legs at the Olympia level. They were huge. By contrast, Fred Hatfield was the first man to ever squat 1,000 lbs., but Fred's legs wouldn't turn heads at a local bodybuilding show. Similarly, Tom Platz was never, ever going to be able to squat 1,000 lbs.

Here's the thing: Tom "used squats" in his leg training, while Fred trained for 1RM squat limit strength. Tom's focus was training the muscles, not the movement. Fred trained for the execution of the movement. Tom's goal was to stimulate his muscles for growth. Fred's goal was to make a barbell move from A to B.

The funny thing here is that Fred Hatfield *himself*, at the time, said to me once, "There is never a reason to do single rep lifts in bodybuilding training."

Fred also told me, "The legs are relatively inactive in the powerlifting-style squat."

This was coming from the first man to squat 1,000 lbs.!

But Fred understood the real principles at work. If anyone should ever have had paradigm blindness toward limit strength training expression, it should have been Fred. But no: he understood the principles on a deeper level.

So, you wonder: if I shouldn't train for pure "strength," or for a huge one-rep max, then how should I train? Do I just add a bunch of reps?

The answer lies in strength density training.

Strength Density Training for Maximum Hypertrophy

If you are a Hardgainer, then development is going to come as a result of strength density training.

This means getting "stronger" at many different rep ranges along the strength curve.

It means that for the Hardgainer, development isn't only about lifting "more." It's about lifting better and lifting smarter.

Yes, lifting "more" will be one result of this kind of program, but it should not be the goal of it. Development is your goal, not how much you can lift. And how much you can lift is seldom an indicator of how much you should lift, within any given workout program.

If you are a Hardgainer you've been told many times that the weights work the muscle, and therefore you need to lift more.

After four decades of experience in this game and studying Hardgainers, I can tell you the opposite is true: it's not the weights that work the muscles; it's the muscles that work the weights.

Read that over again. Twice.

It's about using your muscles to work the weights. The muscles work the weights. The muscles work the weights. I've already repeated it several times in this book. But I do so again! It's that important!

The point isn't "just" to move a weight from point A to point B. The point is to maximally activate the muscle through a full range of motion.

When you engage this reality properly, when you understand it and absorb it, then you can develop your physique maximally.

Look, if you are a true Hardgainer (and especially a natural Hardgainer) you aren't going to compete with the mass monsters dominating the Mr. Olympia stage. Let's be realistic here.

But it also doesn't mean you have to settle for no development at all.

You can absolutely sculpt an enviable physique

that turns heads on the beach, in the gym, and anywhere else.

At my first contest in 1983, I won, but I only weighed in at a scrawny 154 lbs. Only four years later, in 1987, I won the Great Lakes Bodybuilding Championships, and I weighed in on stage at 235 lbs. That is a lot of muscle in a short time. I developed my body and added that muscle by staying true to the principles I'm outlining here. I will provide more of the details below.

I was never the strongest guy in the gym. I learned the hard way, through trial and error, research, and talking with guys who had more experience than me, that I didn't have to be the strongest. I learned the hard way that training with that mindset of "strength first" only left me frustrated or injured. If you are a Hardgainer, you've probably experienced the same thing.

This program is based on what I've learned over the past four decades about how to train for physique development. Once I turned my attention specifically toward you Hardgainers, I've been able to "tweak" what I've learned into a model, a package, and a step-by-step process that just works.

And what's more important, you can have fun doing it. Training should NOT be frustrating. It should be engaging!

Secrets from the Bodybuilding Golden Age

Let's begin with some history.

Some of you reading this will never have heard of Bill Pearl, but he was THE first real superstar in the bodybuilding world.

He wrote Keys to The Inner Universe, and the book still sells well today. Bill won "World's Best Built Man" several times, as well as the Mr. Universe title, and a whole bunch of other impressive fitness and bodybuilding titles.

Bill was also my first real mentor in this industry.

I learned a lot from him and from the bodybuilders of his day, and they themselves had all learned the value of "biofeedback." Real biofeedback comes from this era of bodybuilders. Bill forged his physique in the early years and then again later on with whole body training. And whole body training is part of the Hardgainer Solution when it comes to training.

At a symposium where Bill and I were speaking back in 2005, we were all sitting around at dinner and sharing war stories of the industry. There were a bunch of industry giants sitting there at the table. They all shared the similar story of going to visit Bill and how Bill trained for hours and hours per day. Shyly, Bill admitted that yes, he would train from 3:30 a.m. sometimes till 7:30 a.m. doing whole body workouts and just getting lost in it. Now, yes, absolutely, three to four hours of training per day is probably overtraining and unrealistic for most of us, especially Hardgainers. But it was how Bill trained the intrigued me.

Namely, it was his whole body workouts, combined with how he trained during those workouts, that I realized provided the real key for Hardgainers.

I first met Bill, and encountered the way he trained, back at Muscle Camp in California in 1989.

Muscle Camp for many people was a chance to see and be seen in the mecca of bodybuilding, and in Hollywood as well, for that matter. That is how most people looked at having the privilege of being at, and working at, Muscle Camp.

The whole "Camp" took place at Loyola Marymount University in Los Angeles. We stayed in the dorms. The university's basketball gymnasium was converted into this gigantic training gym, unlike anything else at the time.

Equipment manufacturers would send equipment prototypes to be there, and only there - and everyone wanted to come to Joe Weider's Muscle Camp and work out. Here I was, hired and paid to be there as an expert.

I explained to my bosses there that even though I had to train and teach others through the day there, I actually preferred training alone, when the gym was less busy.

I talked them into giving me a key and I began to work out every morning in what was probably, at the time, the best training facility in the world – just up the street from Muscle Beach, Gold's Gym, and World Gym.

(I remember thinking that I actually had the "key" to the best training facility in the world.)

I got up every morning at, I don't know, about 4:30 a.m., I guess, even though we had Muscle Camp responsibilities until about 11:00 pm every night.

I was always the one to open the gym before 5 a.m., turn on the lights, and have at it. I had a nickname around Muscle Camp and then later at World Gym. They called me the "Crazy Canuck." Joe Gold, World Gym owner, and original founder of Gold's Gym, gave me the nickname and it stuck.

So as fate would have it, here I am opening the gym every morning and "hangin' and bangin'" all by myself in there. Talk about being a kid in a candy store.

One morning as I'm turning on the lights and getting to it, in walks another man along with me. It was Bill Pearl!

You have to keep in mind this gym was enormous in size. Two people could be in there and never even see each other. I got to my business, huffin' and puffin' and leaving a sweat trail that you could use to find me if I were lost.

Eventually I ended up on a piece of equipment Bill was using. I asked if I could work in. He said "sure."

Aside from that I never spoke to him, he never spoke to me: we were just truly "having at it," separately, but together.

He kept an eye on me, and later he joined me for breakfast. We chatted. He seemed impressed that someone as young as me would be in there training alone, and training hard at that. Next morning, before the light of day, at the gym, there I was, and there was Bill, AGAIN. The mutual respect just took off from there. I watched Bill train like an artist – completely connected to the "tools of the trade."

But I noticed he worked his whole body, still by body parts mind you, but he did his whole body in each workout, even on back-to-back days.

Academically and scientifically, this was sacrilege back then. But this was Bill Pearl for crying out loud! So I didn't say anything, and observed in quiet.

A few nights later, we had dinner. We talked about all things training, life, etc. Now, it was obvious that academically and in terms of research, I actually had a better handle on the actual "science" of training. But so what? Bill had the handle on real-world experience and success. And now, all these years later the lessons I learned from Bill Pearl have sparked the foundation for the workouts of The Hardgainer's Solution.

On a similar note I'd like to mention one other icon from the earlier days of the bodybuilding industry.

The late Serge Nubret from France had one of the best physiques of all time. He was famous and notorious for doing very high rep training with what many considered very "light" weights. He also moved at a consistent pace, without ever seeming out of breath, but never sitting to rest either. Serge Nubret seldom did sets of less than 15 to 20 reps – and he had what would still be to this day one of the best physiques of all time. When I spoke to Serge a long, long time ago at FIBO in Europe, he told me he always considered "the pump" to be far more important than the load he used for any given exercise. In fact, he said, if he couldn't feel a pump, then he would make the weight lighter, not heavier.

You can see Serge Nubret in the film *Pumping Iron* where he finished second to Arnold in Mr. Olympia, but ahead of Lou Ferrigno. In fact, if you pay attention to the training sequences in that film, you will witness far more high rep training than low rep "get strong" training. (*Pumping Iron* is also the same film where

Arnold compares the pump to an orgasm.)

Enter Whole Body Training for Hardgainer Success

After decades of observation of Hardgainers, it just seems obvious to me now, that relative to other forms of training, the systemic effects of whole body training are far more anabolic over time, while at the same time having the benefit of being far less risky of the catabolic effects associated with body part training. This is especially so when we're talking about a "natural" trainee who is also a Hardgainer.

The mistake other gurus and pundits make is they focus on how muscles adapt to stress, and then they say "therefore train like this," usually with some strength-based protocol.

They should be seeing the Hardgainer differently. If the Hardgainer's muscles and body responded to simple classic "overload," then any overload program would work for them. These gurus and pundits miss the point that Hardgainers are a special population and training for this group may have to be special as well.

Moreover, you have to look at training in all three realms of time adaptation:

- The **Immediate** effects

- The **Residual** effects

- The **Cumulative** effects

To put it simply, the systemic and *lasting* anabolic effects of Whole Body Training make the most sense if you consider yourself a Hardgainer.

Most books for Hardgainers offer only a tactical approach to training. They'll give you a program that gives you the recovery you need, but at the expense of volume. Others will give you the volume you need to grow, but at the expense of your recovery.

The whole body training protocol here is strategically designed to give you both.

Peripheral Heart Action Training

Another element of this program is Peripheral Heart Action training.

I could get into a long explanation of PHA and its history, but let's keep it simple.

Peripheral Heart Action training is about blood circulating to different areas of the body and different body parts at the same time.

In the HGS program as it appears here, I've tweaked the classical approach to PHA training to fit the Whole Body approach.

Here is what you need to know about why this type of training is so effective for the Hardgainer.

First of all PHA training is NOT "circuit" training. It is purely about blood delivery and exchange. It's about getting a better pump (a more *immediate* effect of training), as well as training the body *over time* to create better and better pumps (the *cumulative* and *residual* effects of training).

This is very efficient for neuromuscular effects and for training the muscles. By mixing up the rep schemes and the targeted body parts in each and every workout, we create greater and enhanced neurological pathways to the muscles, and we increase the response from the muscles as well.

Think of it as creating "off-ramps" and "collector lanes" for busy highways. By using whole body workouts and PHA training, we are doing the same thing. We're increasing blood flow to the muscles as we train, and *at the same time* we're training ourselves to get better at increasing blood flow to the muscles in the future.

Not many experts look at this element of training, especially when it comes Hardgainers, but I have always considered it one of the most important aspects of training.

Muscle fiber recruitment is already a central problem for the Hardgainer. But by combining body part targets in biplexes and triplexes, as well as doing structured whole body training, we go a long way toward remedying this.

In other words, Hardgainers still need to do targeted single joint body part training, but they must do it in a way that enhances neural efficiency, and that's why we're combining PHA training with whole body workouts.

The whole body PHA workouts outlined below accomplish this important effect. Once again, what is so ESSENTIAL when designing programs for Hardgainers is that muscle fiber recruitment is a *neural* event, NOT a muscular one. When we make this a priority for the Hardgainer, we go a long way toward solving the Hardgainer problem!

One final point to make regarding PHA training is to not confuse it with metabolic training. For the Hardgainer, PHA training is essential and makes sense, but this does NOT mean working in ongoing oxygen debt (i.e., breathing heavily, starting the next set while still short of breath, and so on). I'll discuss this more in the Rules of Application section of the program itself.

The Rep Schemes That Will Make You Grow

As I've already indicated, this is a whole body program that uses PHA training. But it is also **a reps-based program** and not a load-based program.

It's the rep schemes that drive this program and make it work.

If you glance at the list of workouts, you will see rep schemes of *five, eight to 12, 12 to 15, 15 to 20,* and *20.* These are the rep schemes necessary for *"surfing the curve"* of muscle development. The two most important rep schemes in the above schemes are the five-rep scheme and the 15 to 20- and 20-rep schemes.

The **five-rep scheme** represents the exercise or exercises in the workout where you will target lifting the heaviest weight for that exercise. (But never going to failure.)

The **high rep schemes of 20** are all about cadence and muscle "pump" to gorge the muscles with blood using the selected exercise.

For the Hardgainer, the five-rep scheme should be used sparingly; the 15 to 20, and 20-rep scheme should be the foundation of the program. If unsure, always lean towards the higher rep schemes!

This is likely the opposite of what you've been told regarding lift heavy weight and get stronger. Yes, absolutely, we need to target the higher threshold motor units that a five-rep scheme can target, but we need to do so in a more intelligent way. And we need to do it with proper frequency and in the context of what the overall training effect will be, once you consider the full program (other exercises in that particular complex, other complexes in that day's workout, other workouts that week, and so on.)

Therefore, the more often you train this program, the less you employ the five-rep scheme within a workout and the more you stay at the higher rep schemes of 15 to 20, and 20, as outlined in the workouts.

This is a very important point not to be overlooked!

The more you work out, the less you use the five-rep scheme, and the more you use the higher rep scheme!

This program is made up of workouts, which include three-sequence series of biplexes and triplexes that, over the course of a single workout, target all the major body parts: legs, back, chest, shoulders, biceps, and triceps. They all get hit each and every workout.

Abs exercises are included at the end of each workout and are mostly just to keep the area tight and engaged and to continue the PHA element of the overall training strategy.

Exercise selection, while still important, is not nearly as important in this program as are the rep schemes I've outlined above. This means if your gym is busy, or you don't have the equipment, you can sub in another exercise for that body part... as long as it fits the general program outline, and as long as you follow the rep schemes!

For instance, if the exercise calls for a single side at a time exercise, then you would sub with an exercise that is also the same body part and is also single side at a time. Use your head. For example, you could sub a one-arm preacher curl for a one-arm concentration curl, or you could sub a one-leg leg press with a single-leg lunge. And so on.

Also, even though the exercises are not as important as the rep schemes, I've still outlined a tremendous number of workouts where exercise sequencing and rep schemes fit really well together. **So you would be wise to follow these workouts' protocols as written as much as possible. If in doubt, follow the program. Don't tweak for the sake of tweaking.**

Because this is Whole Body Training, the application potential is limitless, and this makes this program very easy to adapt to real life.

"How Many Days Per Week Should I Train?"

Should you train five days per week? Three? *All seven?*

Short answer: it depends.

At first, if you are a true Hardgainer, you may

want to go every other day with the workouts. But this program is flexible, and these workouts can be done as few as three times per week, and as often as seven days per week, as long as you follow the *Rules of Application* outlined below.

In particular: the more days per week that you train, the higher your rep schemes! As you move from training three to four times per week to five to seven, you should adjust the rep schemes so that the five rep exercises become eight to 10 rep exercises, or 12 to 15, or even 15 to 20, and so on.

You could go two or three days on, with a day off – or work out five days in a row and take weekends off. This program has a very flexible application and it *will* work, as long as you stick to its rules of application, and you *listen to your own biofeedback*. Are you feeling over-trained? Dial it back. Adjust the rep schemes upwards.

I mentioned above that recovery is an incredibly important element of this program. Most people neglect two kinds of recovery for the Hardgainer: **inter-workout** (between workouts) and **intra-workout** (within the workout).

The overall program design, whole body

workouts, and sets and reps approach already takes care of inter-workout recovery. But within the workout is where most Hardgainers go wrong and end up pushing against their own recovery. This will set the Hardgainer back. So here we need to talk about oxygen debt and pace.

The Right Workout Pace For Success

In some of my MET programs, and even my innervation training programs, I focus on oxygen debt and workout pace.

But I also always focus on context.

Because of everything I've just outlined, for these workouts *you want to work at a comfortable pace and never push the pace*. There is no rush to get from the one exercise in a sequence to the next. For the Hardgainer, and for this program in particular, you want to keep oxygen debt in check.

Once the workout starts, you should never be too out of breath, and you should be able to keep moving without needing to sit down to rest. However, on high rep leg exercises, sometimes you may get deeper into oxygen debt and this is understandable. But other than a few exceptions you should be moving at a comfortable and reasonable pace where labored breathing is okay and expected, but panting or needing to sit down for more than a few seconds means you've overextended your recovery capacity.

So gauge your oxygen debt accordingly, and do not push the pace of your workouts. That's not the point of this program! **This is a muscle and physique development program; it is NOT a conditioning program.**

Hardgainers need to learn to focus on one main area. And for you this means building and developing the physique. Conditioning concerns can come later or in another form. So you never want to be too deep in an oxygen debt and you want to gauge this biofeedback indicator as intra-workout recovery. This is why certain exercises are continued from one sequence into the next. For instance, often Bulgarian Split Squats are only done *one side per round* in order to make sure the targeted muscle is engaged, while also ensuring not getting too deep into oxygen debt and affecting *intra*-workout recovery and training pace.

The Importance of Undertraining.
(Yes, _under_training.)

If you're a Hardgainer, you may have felt you needed to train hard enough to induce an adaptive response, but as a Hardgainer you may *also* have never properly *recovered* from the harder or heavier workouts. It's a problem of different variables being in conflict with each other.

So you get "some" results or "a little" progress up front, but the lack of recovery kept you from really developing your physique beyond an initial honeymoon period. This program solves the issue is many ways.

First, by never going too far—or at all—into oxygen debt, you have optimal recovery *within* the workout.

Next, because you are doing Whole Body and body part training, you are not over-stimulating any one body part beyond recovery capacity. By combining attention to *intra*-workout recovery capacity and *inter*-workout recovery capacity, you can finally train consistently enough to accrue an ongoing adaptive response and create an optimum internal biochemical and hormonal environment for muscle growth and adaptation.

Moreover, because of the focus on high reps and pumping cadence, recovery capacity from this type of training is also enhanced. All of these things are very important considerations for the Hardgainer. And they are well beyond the faulty logic that you've been told that 'just train for strength and development will come.' You need to erase that advice from your memory.

But the key here is an emphasis in "*undertraining*" all around.

Yes, you heard that right: undertraining.

You have to remember you are a Hardgainer for a number of reasons. How the "champions" (the ones you might envy) built their bodies really *doesn't apply to you* and your Hardgainer physiology. Also, the ways in which champions use a litany of performance enhancing drugs to create their physiques really doesn't apply to you and your physiology either.

So you need to stop paying attention to what these various individuals and groups do to train their bodies. You simply do not fit into that demographic if you describe yourself as a Hardgainer.

So you need to heed this point:

You want to always be a bit undertrained.

Well the question becomes *how* do you do that, and what does it feel like?

- First, you want to keep account of your oxygen debt.

- You never want your breathing to get into the panting zone, or the "sit down for two minutes to recover" zone.

- For exercise cadence, you do NOT want to do any exercise "explosively." The Hardgainer must strip everything down to its essentials.

- You will work with a pumping cadence most of the time and "stretch the muscle with resistance."

- And then on heavy five-rep exercises, where applicable, like squats and benches and overhead presses, you will move the weight purposefully but slowly, always under control.

You undertrain by always selecting a weight you can do comfortably for the reps indicated and *NEVER going to failure.*

Leave at least a two to four rep performance window as your guide when selecting what load to use.

The final indicator of proper undertraining is to leave the gym after each workout feeling, subjectively, like you had a *good* workout, *but that you could have done just a bit more.*

This means you are not working beyond your own recovery capacity. Don't worry: over time you will build up your work capacity by working in this way.

So, leaving the gym feeling like you could have done more is actually a **good sign** if you are a Hardgainer. Remember always that as a Hardgainer you are part of a unique population, so unique rules and principles must apply as well. Furthermore, as a

Hardgainer you have to learn to look and think long-term, and not just "right now." Each workout in the HGS program is like a feeder system to the next workout, and then to the next month's workouts. This obviously won't work if you burn yourself out in the short term.

So, undertraining a bit should be your mantra.

And you do this by never going to failure on any exercise – moving at a comfortable but not exhausting pace in your workout – never getting too far into oxygen debt – and leaving the gym feeling like you had a good workout, but that you could have done more. These are the ESSENTIAL biofeedback indicators you want to use within and between workouts to gauge your recovery, your consistency, and your progress. So once again I remind you that you can let go of focusing on 'how heavy' you lift and pay more attention to these other far more important performance parameters.

A note on deadlifts:

You will not see deadlifts or leg curl exercises on this program. We want to strip things down to the key essentials for the Hardgainer. The deadlift is an exercise with far too high an injury risk, and it doesn't target any one area very well. For these two reasons, I've left it out. If you are a trainee who really loves the deadlift, then you can put in the RDL variation, but use it sparingly if you do. And you would use it as a back exercise.

Still, I would prefer it be left out altogether on this program. Leg curls can have some value, but they are mostly for strengthening deceleration effects, and if you are a Hardgainer there isn't much value in them in a Whole Body Program. In terms of hamstring development, as a Hardgainer you will get enough hamstring involvement with the leg press, lunge, squat variations and bent over movements prescribed in the program. Again, if you wanted to use a leg curls exercise, do so sparingly and keep reps in the higher rep zones – but for the Hardgainer, it's really not called for in this program.

Conclusion

The consistent advice to trainees to just "lift more" makes no sense for the Hardgainer, if you break it down.

Being able to lift substantially more is a training effect, yes, but it is also about muscle fiber types an individual may or may not have and may or may not be able to activate well. My question to the Hardgainer who is told to "lift to get strong," and has been doing so for years without success, is this: "If you could get optimum development by training this way, wouldn't you already be there?"

Training for sheer 1RM strength is simply not going to develop your body if you are a Hardgainer.

Not enough attention gets paid to recovery capacity and the internal biochemical and hormonal environments of the Hardgainer. All these Internet experts are focusing on what kind of stimulus YOU the Hardgainer should be under. But few, if any of them, look at what your recovery needs are, and this includes your day-to-day recovery between workouts, as well as the type of recovery you need between exercises within a single training session.

This is also a fundamental mistake when experts only look at principles of muscle adaptation, without considering the trainee as a whole person and where their particular obstacles to development may lie.

Finally, the last problem for the Hardgainer worth mentioning lies with you as the trainee.

To be brutally honest: most Hardgainers simply do not stick with sound training protocol long enough to get a permanent effect on their physiques. Because you are a Hardgainer, you keep looking for some "holy grail" program to get you to the promised land of physique development.

More than likely this has led you to bouncing from one program to another, without ever giving a single good program enough time to work. I call this the "pinballing" habit. (I'll address this in a later section.)

The program I have outlined below requires a minimum one-year commitment if you really want to start accruing serious muscle development.

I cannot stress this enough.

I've given you enough workouts that you could work out every single day until you've gone through the program, then rinse, repeat, and that would give you six months of training each and every day.

You'll also get rules for adjusting and creating your own workouts, so you can keep going and, as I say, "keep the program alive," so that each time you step into the gym you're fresh, excited, and constantly improving.

Okay. Enough of that. Let's get into the nitty gritty of your training.

Part 2.

The Hardgainer's Workout and Training Solution

A Note on the Most Neglected Part of Training

The most neglected, underappreciated, and misapplied element of a training session is almost always to do with a proper, effective and efficient **warm-up.**

Of all the people who venture here to train with me in my home workout dungeon, I'd say 99% make the mistake of rushing through the warm-up, and they do it without paying attention to the *quality* of the warm-up.

But the quality and efficiency of your warm-up ALWAYS leads to how optimized your workout performance will or will not be. Almost all modern trainees I've seen in action underestimate a proper warm-up. You don't *ever* rush warm-ups or physical rehearsal for your training session. And of the two elements of workouts discussed here (warm-ups, and cool-downs,) warm-ups are far more important when it comes to getting the most out of a training session. So while post-workout stretching is optional, efficient and proper pre-workout "warm-ups" should ALWAYS be considered as an integral part of any workout.

Let's talk about what makes a quality proper warm-up to get you primed for a quality training session.

Warm-up Sequencing & Execution

When it comes to warm-ups, the first question to address is, "What will I actually be doing in the next hour?" In other words, what is the workout emphasis: with what exercise are you starting with upper body, or lower body? These considerations should influence the 'General Preparation Phase' (GPP) and specific physical rehearsal.

GPP, or, General Preparation Phase

- The General Preparation Phase should last anywhere from seven to 15 minutes or so. There is a primary emphasis on knees, hips, and shoulders, then a secondary emphasis on ankles, elbows and wrists. Notice the emphasis is joint-connected, not necessarily muscle-oriented. After primary and secondary "emphasis" then the "focus" should be on ROM, multiple planes, unloading where necessary. Therefore, think in terms of warm-up as moving, reaching, bending, balancing, rotating COM (Center of Mass) as in "twisting" (usually involving the hips/waist).

• The rule to remember is to warm up to stretch, and to NEVER stretch to warm up.

• Why? For optimal results, flexibility exercises in the warm-up should be active, that is, involving movement to facilitate the excitation of the nervous system to create a readiness for movement. The purpose of stretching in a warm-up is neural activation. Passive and static forms of stretching have a calming effect. That is appropriate for a cool down, but NOT for getting ready to train. Static stretching is inappropriate for a warm-up.

Note: Static stretching can be counterproductive if placed before a workout requiring explosiveness, speed or agility (that doesn't leave many types of training that aren't already stretch dependent e.g. yoga!) Immediately after static stretching, the muscles are less responsive to stimulation, and co-ordination is thrown off. Static stretches interfere with the activity of tendon reflexes.

- The amount of work required to maintain flexibility is significantly less than the amount of time required to develop it…. Arm swings, leg swings, trunk rotations, reaches, and bending stimulate blood flow and wake up the nervous system.

- So the overall emphasis is also nervous system, and cardiorespiratory activation, in terms of mild core temperature connection. Think in very "literal" terms when it comes to "warming up." The commonly performed sitting on a bike or walking on a treadmill or doing light sets of leg extensions and other ideas are NOT warming up for a workout, or preparing for resistance training.

- Too much emphasis is placed on raising core temperature and heart rate in the warm-up. The main physiological objective is **neural**

activation – getting everything firing to prepare for the more intense work to follow.

• Try to stay away from stationary bikes and steppers as part of the warm-up. These machines encourage a restricted range of motion, in that they shorten the psoas muscles, which could have negative effects on the subsequent workout.

• Unloading the knees, and including regular full squatting in workouts, not only helps the knees, but increases and aids the mobility of pelvic and hip joints.

Integrated Warm-up/Specific Physical Rehearsal

• Near the end of GPP, start to warm-up specific muscles that will actually be the main focus of the workout or the first exercise. So, therefore you "**integrate**" into the warm-up, more and more specific exercises of lighter sets, and higher, slower reps of the actual exercise that will come first in your workout. This is called "physical rehearsal." And you can from there progressively increase load, ROM, intensity, etc., without yet doing an actual "work set." Sometimes nothing more than two to three sets need to be used in physical rehearsal. Physical rehearsal need not last more than five to seven minutes, depending on the load variant that will be implemented.

Cool-Down Emphasis

- The post-workout cool-down should last a minimum of 10 minutes, and up to 30 minutes at the high range.

- The goal is to stretch muscles, especially the muscles worked in that training session. At the same time, the goal is **not** to *over*-stretch muscles.

- The cool down is **not** a workout, and should not feel like one. If it does… you are over-stretching. Cool down is **NOT** a Yoga class. Cooling down is all about initiating recovery, and relieving workout-induced muscle stiffness.

- The cool-down emphasis should target, most specifically: hips, glutes, hamstrings, low back, shoulders and kinetic chains. These should be the main emphasis of every cool down session.

- Take a posture or position and hold each one for a slow count of 12 to 25 (or four deep breaths) before moving to a new posture or position. You should be able to feel the tension in the muscles release as you hold the stretch. So take the position or posture only to the point where you feel the tension, and hold at that position for release. This is called your "edge."

- Use any combination of stretches from a standing or floor position. There should be a minimum of five to 10 sequences per cool down session.

- It's ok to mix them up as well. You can stick to a primary routine, or you can change it daily or every few days. Don't get stuck on thinking in terms of "right" or "wrong."

And remember: "warm up to stretch; we do not stretch to warm up."

Important General Notes

- Warm up to stretch, do not stretch to warm up. Static stretching is for *post*-workout. Dynamic stretching via 'warming up' is for before the workout.

- Warming up before a workout primarily serves as 'physical rehearsal' and neural activation for the intense exercise to come. As well it serves to lubricate joints, increase blood flow to appropriate places and prepare the cardio-respiratory system.

- Stiff muscles are the result of inactivity, sedentary lifestyle and even aging. Of all of these, the first two contribute the most to problems.

- Stretching serves to develop key body awareness. This is crucial in learning and appreciating "biofeedback" which is such an important term in the Abel Body Methodology.

Stretching totally cold muscles can cause injury, as can over-stretching. Stretch after training, and remember it is not meant to be a workout or to feel "hard." Stretching should never be painful; if it is, you are testing yourself and going past your "edge" point.

The Benefits of Post-Workout Stretching

Too few people actually devote time to *post*-workout stretching. You need to start viewing it as an optional part of the workout, if you have time.

- Stretching is merely the activity of contracting and releasing muscles to lengthen, strengthen, and lubricate them – and return them to their original length (known as viscoelasticity).

- Flexibility, coordination and balance diminish as you age – stretching can slow down this effect and preserve this healthy state.

- Most people lose rotational ability of joints (e.g. shoulders, neck, etc.) as they age.

- By strengthening weaker muscles in a kinetic chain, and lengthening them with stretching, your posture improves.

- Regular stretching leads to increased circulation and this blood supply effect serves the body in many healthy ways. Over time you will experience a sense of rejuvenation.

• Stretching can relieve many symptoms of stress, not just physically-induced by training, but life-stressors as well. Stretching is shown to improve or even eliminate back and neck pain, arthritis, digestive issues, insomnia, general fatigue or malaise, and a weakened immune system (this one because of the benefit of increased circulation mentioned above.)

• Now, keep in mind also that body part weight training is, in essence, all about training a muscle through a full range of motion – so this does have some added benefits already depending on the program and the level of development of the trainee.

• Stretching also serves that key Abel Body principle of mind/body awareness. Stretching draws your attention to your body and your body to your mental awareness. The pay-offs of this are rich.

- Stretching serves to realign the body. Many forces of gravity and daily activities can lead to structural misalignment over time.

- A general rule of thumb is that you should stretch a minimum of three days per week, but the harder and more frequently you train, the more you should stretch, if you have the time. So, at the high end of performance, you should stretch as often as you train. Like diet and training – consistency is everything.

- Breathing deeply (four deep breaths) for each stretch is advisable. But not all stretches lend to easy and deep breathing. That's ok. Just try to hold a stretch for 30 seconds.

- Your muscles and joints should never be locked into place. There should always be a certain sense and feeling of "relaxed" in the targeted stretch position.

- **HIPS:** Stretching "resets" the body. If you don't stretch after intense workouts or exercise, you'll experience a "domino" effect of symptoms. Consider the domino effect of the most common point of tightness and largest joint in the body – the hips. The hips can make your back tight, pull your pelvis forward, roll your thighs outward, and lead to pressure and pain in both your lower back and your knees. Rigid hips can change your posture, inhibit movement, and tighten groin muscles, the hip rotators, hip flexors and other muscle extensors in the area. These imbalances can "refer" to other areas creating pain – most notably, low back stiffness and pain and decreased ROM.

- **HAMSTRINGS:** Can you bend over and touch your toes? Do you slouch? If your answers are no and yes respectively, you have tight hamstrings. Tight hamstrings can also "refer" pain and stress onto other joints, including the hips, the knees and the low back. Are you starting to see a connected pattern here? Tight hamstrings restrict the extension of your hips. Tight hamstrings can lead to you rounding your back and slouching and this can lead to – you guessed it, tight and stressed shoulder or neck area. Weak hamstrings can also create more stress in the quadriceps and this imbalance can lead to poor posture, poor balance, poor kinesthetic awareness, etc. Hamstrings are also directly tied to core muscles. Therefore stretching the hamstrings in a variety of ways is actually mild work for the abs/core as well. Any Yoga practitioner knows that.

- Combined, a lack of elasticity in both your hamstrings and hips inhibits your ability to bend forward. This leads to a tight back, and makes the back area more susceptible to injury such as disc herniation, etc.

- **KNEES:** like hips and shoulders, your knees typically lose their ROM both as you age, and as a result of a lot of sitting and the modern sedentary lifestyle. Stretching helps restore some mobility.

- **LOWER BACK:** As shown above, back issues are often the result of any combination of other related problems that end up playing out in back pain or injury. Such issues for example are often the result of tension between your abdominal muscles and the hamstrings. It is foolish to just try to segment both these areas for "strength training" without realizing that the ongoing tightness of both areas can cause tension between them, resulting in back issues. Weak torso muscles of the core, anterior or posterior, the ones that attach to the spine, can be major contributors to back pain. Constantly riding, or running or treadmill work to "begin" a workout shortens and tightens muscles of the psoas and can actually contribute to injury or stiffness and tension over time.

Rotating, extending, and aligning your spinal column – via dynamic motion and static stretching post-workout, increases circulation of blood and oxygen in your muscles, and more importantly, hydrates the discs of the spine and neck. All of this serves to alleviate stiffness.

how to
FOLLOW
the HGS PROGRAM

Performing Complexes

As you look through the programs you will notice that all of the exercises are grouped into either groups of two or three exercises like 'a' and 'b' (for two exercises), or 'a', 'b' & 'c' (for three). There are only a few exceptions where there is a single exercise not performed in a complex or superset of some sort.

These two or three individual exercises are grouped together by number. These groups are known as "complexes" and the idea is that exercise a), exercise b) and exercise c) of that complex are performed back to back. Performing all three (or all two) of those exercises constitutes one set for a complex.

After a set, you rest until you are ready to repeat the set again, and ready to perform the two or three exercises again back to back. You repeat the total amount of sets prescribed before moving on to the next group of exercises (i.e. the next complex) and you execute the next complex in the same fashion.

I will illustrate with an example from "Workout 1" below:

WORKOUT 1.

Exercise	Sets X Reps
1a) DB or BB Squats	5 X 5
1b) DB Incline Press	5 X 8-10
1c) DB or BB Upright Rows	5 X 20
2a) Pull-downs Behind the Head	4 X 12-15
2b) 2 Arm DB Curl	4 X 20
3a) One-arm DB triceps extension	4 X 5-6
3b) Any sit-up or leg raise variation	4 X 20

Exercise 1a), 1b) and 1c) represent your first complex. You perform them all back to back, and at an even pace, for the number of reps prescribed for each of the three exercises. In other words, you perform five reps of dumbbell or barbell squats, then immediately you perform eight to 10 reps of dumbbell incline press, then immediately you

perform 20 reps of dumbbell or barbell upright rows, then you rest, and that's one set. You have four more sets of this complex, for a total of five. Then you move on to Complex 2.

You'll figure out the right pace as you go. Remember I said not to rush. This isn't a conditioning workout. Take as much of a break as you require between each movement in order to keep the pace comfortable and not totally exhausting. Don't just watch the clock. Read your own biofeedback.

When you have completed five sets of the three exercises in Complex 1, you move on to the second complex, which includes both 2a) and 2b), and you perform this complex in the same fashion. When you have completed all four sets of the second complex, move on to the third complex, including both 3a) and 3b), and you execute in the same fashion as the first two complexes for all four sets prescribed.

This should adequately explain "complexes" to those of you who may not have done them before.

Occasional Overlapping Sets for Split-Leg or Split-Arm Exercises

This is the most "complicated" part of the workout program, but it's actually very simple, and you could probably skip this section and know what the workouts mean. But I'll explain anyway, just so it's here for reference.

As I mentioned in the workout pace section, occasionally you will perform some exercises only one side at a time, and therefore in order to hit both sides for the required number of sets, an exercise in one complex will have to continue on or "spillover" into the next complex.

Here is an example, using **Workout 22**.

Look in particular at 2c) and 3c) on the following page.

WORKOUT 22.

Exercise	Sets X Reps
1a) One-arm DB Rows	5 X 15-20
1b) One-arm DB triceps extensions	5 X 15
2a) Flat DB Bench Press	4 X 5
2b) BW Bulgarian Split Squat*	4 X 15-20
3a) Cable Rear Delts	4 X 15-20
3b) One-arm Zottman Curls	4 X 12-15ES
3c) Continue BW Bulgarian Split Squat from Complex 2	

* Do only one leg per round in complex 2b). Therefore, you would do right leg on the first round of exercise 2b) and left leg on the second round of exercise 2b). So to complete all four sets of Bulgarian Split Squats, this exercise will "spill" into Complex 3.

To clarify how this spillover works, here's what the entire first complex would look like in execution:

5 reps of Flat DB Bench Press
15 to 20 reps of BW Bulgarian Split Squat (right leg)
Rest.

5 reps of Flat DB Bench Press
15 to 20 reps of BW Bulgarian Split Squat (left leg)
Rest.

5 reps of Flat DB Bench Press
15 to 20 reps of BW Bulgarian Split Squat (right leg)
Rest.

5 reps of Flat DB Bench Press
15 to 20 reps of BW Bulgarian Split Squat (left leg)

At this point, you've done four sets of Flat DB Bench Press. But for each individual leg, you've only done two sets (two for the right, two for the left). Therefore, you continue the Bulgarian Split Squats into the next complex until you've done all four sets for both legs for that exercise.

The third complex would thus look like this in execution:

15 to 20 reps Cable Rear Delts
12 to 15 reps One-arm Zottman Curls
15 to 20 reps of BW Bulgarian Split Squat (right leg)
rest

15 to 20 reps Cable Rear Delts
12 to 15 reps One-arm Zottman Curls
15 to 20 reps of BW Bulgarian Split Squat (left leg)
rest

15 to 20 reps Cable Rear Delts
12 to 15 reps One-arm Zottman Curls
15 to 20 reps of BW Bulgarian Split Squat (right leg)
rest

15 to 20 reps Cable Rear Delts
12 to 15 reps One-arm Zottman Curls
15 to 20 reps of BW Bulgarian Split Squat (left leg)
rest

By the end of this complex, you've now hit both the right leg and the left leg for four sets each.

Whenever a spillover like this this occurs, it's all accounted for in the program, and there will be a note of it.

For the sake of being 100% exhaustive here, to see what it looks like when you don't continue on with a split leg or split arm exercise, look at the first complex in the workout above. There is no note about splitting things up, or continuing things on into the next complex, so in the first complex you perform both arms for One-arm DB Rows and both arms for One-arm Triceps Extensions each and every set. In other words, one "set" of the first complex looks like this:

20 reps one-arm DB Row (left arm)
20 reps one-arm DB row (right arm)
5 reps one-arm triceps extension (left arm)
5 reps one-arm triceps extension (right arm)
Rest, repeat

Because you are completing both arms each and every set, there is no need for "spillover" for either exercise.

the
RULES *of* APPLICATION

- As stated above you *never train to failure* on any of the exercises. By your own subjective interpretation, leave a two to four rep window between your last rep and failure.

- Train at an even but controllable pace.

- That is, you never want to get too far into oxygen debt. Even when switching between exercises within a complex there is no "hurry" to rush the pace from exercise "a" to "b" or "c." Your focus is to be challenged by meeting the rep ranges called for and NOT by the pace of your workout. So when in doubt, slow the pace so you can select a challenging load for the reps indicated.

- Once you begin the workout, you should seldom need to sit down and rest between sets. If you do, it shouldn't be for more than a few seconds to half a minute or so. If you need longer, you are going too fast or training too close to failure. This distinction will help you to gauge your intra-workout biofeedback cues.

- You can train up to seven days per week with this program or as few as three days per week. You can tweak the workout format to fit well into any real-life scenario or lifestyle.

- You will make an integrated warm-up a part of the workout. Therefore you can still be doing warm-up exercises like arm swings and leg swings even though you have begun the workout. This is explained in the video and the warm-up section.

- There are five sets of exercise Sequence 1 in every workout; since it is the first sequence, an extra warm-up prep set makes sense.

- Workouts should not last longer than 45 to 50 minutes. And for the Hardgainer, this is also important, because length of workout will affect recovery.

- Exercises can be substituted and changed for other similar exercises as long as they target the same body part in the same way. So, one-arm or one-leg exercises can be subbed for any other one-leg or one-arm exercises – and the same is true for any traditional exercise. But you do NOT change the rep schemes. This is a reps-based program. And the reps application within the workouts is the most important thing.

- *Within the rep schemes,* you are free to do classical pyramiding – where you increase weight each set – or descending pyramids where you do less weight but higher reps each set – or you can stay with a "constant weight" if it "feels" right to you. As long as you do not violate the reps called for, this is where your freedom in day-to-day training lies. For instance, if the rep scheme listed is 12 to 15, or 15 to 20 – you may want to do your first set with a lighter weight for a higher number of reps. Then, you may want to increase the weight and aim for the lower reps listed in the next set. Similarly, for the usual four sets, you could also do two sets at the lower rep range and finish with two sets at the higher reps range. Or you could stay with all four sets at one end or the other for the called for rep range. In other words, as long as you stay within the rep schemes called for – you can vary "how" you choose to do that from set to set. You could start with the lower rep range and heavier weight for the first set, and go progressively lighter each set as well. As long as you follow all the other rules – these are good variations to keep in mind during each workout.

- I suggest frequent time off as well. If you follow this program closely, and you're hitting your workouts with intensity, and you're working out five days or more per week, then I suggest you take one week off training and diet every 12 weeks. If you are a trainee who follows this protocol four days or less per week, then I suggest you take one week off training and diet every 16 weeks. This is all a part of serving your body by making rest and recuperation (long term, not just short term) a key component of adaptive response moving forward.

All set? I'm going to discuss your diet next, but you can also turn to the Complete List of HGS Workouts to see the workouts themselves.

Part 3.

The Hardgainer's Diet Solution

Training Your Metabolism For Success

A lot has been made about how the Hardgainer should diet to put on muscle. You've likely heard it all: Everything from "bulk up as much as you can" to "get ripped and lean but put on muscle at the same time," and everything in between.

But what is "true" for the truly Hardgainer? This is a tough question, and the answer is tricky.

I've been dealing with Hardgainers for decades and there has <u>never</u> been one easy "one size fits all" approach to dieting for the Hardgainer. The individual was always the exception and every single Hardgainer I have Coached had something unique about him or her compared to the next Hardgainer – especially when it came to metabolism.

Let me repeat: there are no *"one size fits all"* approaches to dieting for the Hardgainer.

However, there *are* some general considerations that remain true across the board, and we need to discuss them.

First, you need to let go of unrealistic expectations. If you've never had "six-pack abs" – then don't try dieting to get them at the same time you "say" you want to develop your body. These are often completely different goals. Development should take precedence. Stop listening to ads that tell you that you can gain 25 lbs. of muscle and get ripped at the same time. I've never seen that actually happen to a Hardgainer (either with my own clients or others'), and I've been in this game at the highest levels for four decades! You need to be realistic.

Now, while diet can indeed help you as a Hardgainer, it is not nearly as important as the right program and meeting your recovery needs from training. Your diet does not need to be too complicated. Simple is ALWAYS better. So stop worrying about any marketing nonsense you may hear regarding complicated formulas for putting on muscle while "getting lean."

Furthermore, forget about all this nonsense of pre, peri, and post workout nutrition. With the Hardgainers workouts solutions your workouts will be too short for any of that to matter.

It is overall calories balance to support recovery and growth that matters. And this must be viewed over the long haul and not in short term "windows" that are more marketing rubbish than reality. Having said that... taking in more calories than you need probably makes good sense for the Hardgainer. I consider it as kind of an insurance policy so your body stays in an anabolic state that will not only support recovery, but stimulate growth as well.

The problem with this idea is the message it sends. None of this implies 'bulking up' in the classic sense, or deliberately overfeeding yourself. *You have to train your metabolism and support it as well.*

For the Hardgainer, simply overfeeding yourself is not supporting your metabolism. You need to coax your metabolism along and how to do this will be outlined in the biofeedback section. You never just want to add "scale weight" for the sake of adding scale weight. Any extra body fat you add that is not "functional weight" merely becomes a mechanical drag for you in your workouts – negatively impacting your workout's stimulation and artificially creating greater recovery demands. Moreover, I've had so many Hardgainers in the past think that bulking up meant more muscle only to find out when they dieted all that new and extra fat off – they were right back where they started. So never let the scale confuse you as to what real "progress" is either. *But you do have to "feed a metabolism" in order to optimize it.*

This means that frequent small feedings through the day makes sense – especially if you are a Hardgainer. You also want to make sure, that of these frequent feedings, protein and carbs make up the major portion of your meals. No Hardgainer on the planet will get anywhere with low carbs diets, intermittent fasting, carb cycling, and the rest of the nonsense that passes for know-how on the Internet.

The SIMPLE Calorie Formula

Now, as much as I hate 'formulas' because of how misleading they become... we need to start *somewhere*. So we are going to work with a simple starting formula and work concentrically out from there, by discussing biofeedback as well. The important thing here is to see this formula only as a starting point. It is not some bible-like dictation with no variation. It is merely a starting reference point from which to begin. Here is the starting formula.

Current bodyweight in kilos X 24

OR

Current bodyweight in pounds X 0.45, then that X 24

This is a simple formula that should give you a starting reference point to where your metabolism currently is. This means it should be easy for you to eat within the calories range provided by this formula. So, for instance – for myself right now – I weigh about 215 lbs.

If I apply the formula for pounds then it is 215 lbs. X 0.45, which equals 96.75. And when I multiply that number by 24 I get 2,322 calories, which of course I would round off at 2,300 calories.

And this is just a *starting reference point* formula to determine '*about*' where most metabolisms will be if they are functional and healthy, and haven't been off-set by sabotaging diet practices – a few of which are mentioned above. So, apply the formula above – whatever your preference may be for pounds or kilos. Look at where it leaves you. Go to the diet-strategy section from here to look at similar weight charts and diet-example breakdowns as well.

Optimizing Your Metabolism Even Further

My suggestion for optimizing metabolism as well as for cosmetic advantage (because who doesn't want that?) is to follow this example, to start.

- Use a five meals per day approach.

- Break meals down to a 40/40/20 (in general) approach. This means about 40% protein, 40% carbs, and 20% healthy fats. But of course these numbers can vary. There is no need to be "married to" these macro guidelines.

- Of the carbs portion 20 to 40% of these carbs 'could be' composed of fibrous carbs, but healthy, protein-sparing starch carbs are the priority.

- Protein choices should include lean healthy animal proteins for at least three of the five meals, while nuts, seeds and legumes could be used as alternative sources as well.

- Healthy fats are listed below as well.

Now, this is just a "starting reference." Remember, there are no magic diet-strategy formulas for gaining muscle development. This is merely a starting guide – You are not "right or wrong" if you veer away from it a bit in any given direction. To think so is just fitness industry nonsense, trying to create rocket science where needless complication should be removed.

How (and When) to Add in Extra Calories

As I mentioned above it makes good sense for the hard-gainer to take in some extra calories above your actual needs. But you must train your metabolism to do so. And this is much simpler than you may think. The point is to get out of short-term thinking when it comes to what "*extra calories*" even suggests. For the hard-gainer I think it makes sense to aim for 200 to 300 calories more per day than the formula above yields.

That doesn't really seem like much, does it?

But 200 calories more per day is actually 73,000 extra calories over the course of the year. (200 X 365) And 300 extra calories per day is actually a whopping 109,500 extra calories over the course of the year. (300 X 365) When viewed over the long-term these '*extra*' calories provide ample support for metabolism while providing an impetus for establishing an internal matrix for building and rebuilding tissue as well.

If you spread these extra daily calories over five meals, then we are talking about 50 to 60 extra calories per meal. In a cooperative and optimized metabolism you are unlikely to even notice 50 to 60 extra calories per meal. It would be a couple bites extra of protein and carbs per meal. Or you could just add the 200 to 300 calories as an extra meal in itself.

This is important because, like I said above, you never want to force feed yourself or eat until you are full. To do so is not metabolically efficient for digestion and absorption and transport of nutrients. There are many options for getting in these extra calories, and it NEVER has to be complicated.

By following such simple inclusions of "extra calories" you are unlikely to put on much extra fat weight, as you would if you just tried to "bulk up."

DIET BIOFEEDBACK
and **RULES** *of* **APPLICATION**

- Start with the above formula for the first week or so and gauge your biofeedback. If you are too hungry between meals or day-to-day, then look to add the 200 to 300 extra calories right away. Find the appropriate diet examples for the calorie levels that suit you in the diets provided below.

- Eat five or six small meals per day, preferably five, but the higher the calories, the more meals suggested.

- You can either space meals out calorically-balanced throughout the day, or gradually taper calories throughout the day. Either approach will work fine. Just be consistent.

- Work within the notion of *"tolerable hunger"* (as described in my book *Beyond Metabolism*). This means you should never feel stuffed or full after any meal. And you should always be hungry in a tolerable way between meals. This indicates adequate digestion of previous meals when mealtime comes around.

- You should be able to achieve and sustain a pump within your workouts. This is an indication of adequate glycogen storage so essential to optimizing metabolism and recovery and growth.

- You should have adequate "energy" to complete the workouts as written, with some energy to spare for your daily activities. This indicates sufficient calorie levels and needs. **HOWEVER**, do not confuse "energy" to complete the workouts with the notion of "motivation." Motivation is mental; energy is physiological. And while they can certainly influence each other, you want to get used to reading biofeedback appropriately.

I also suggest taking at least one meal off the diet as a "free meal" every seven to 10 days. This aids digestion, aids the goal of optimizing metabolism, and makes the diet more psychologically sustainable without derailing progress.

Meal Plan Guidelines

- Eat 'meal 1' when you get up in the morning, or as soon as you practically are able to do so. Eat 'meal 5' (or 'meal 6' if there are six meals listed) just before bed time and then space out remaining meals evenly or as close to evenly as practically possible, between your first and last meal.

- Try to space meals out and do not 'skip' a meal and then add two meals together. Scheduled meal times at regular times of the day are better if practically possible.

- Consume only non-caloric beverages and keep diet soda and coffee consumption in moderation – you should be keeping yourself well hydrated with actual water.

- 'Small salad' refers to a mix of garden-variety vegetables (refer to the 'food-sources' guide) and leafy greens. For example: kale, spinach, cucumber, broccoli, peppers, asparagus, sprouts, etc. For a small salad, **do not** include cheeses, olives, beans or avocado <u>unless</u> specified in the plan. 'Small' refers to about a cup or so in amount.

- Condiments in moderation are fine. These include ketchup, salsa, salt and pepper, etc. (Use salt according to taste – no need to either restrict or over-salt.) Chilies, garlic and all herbs and spices are usually all fine.

- There will be some options for each meal, however choose only **one** of the bulleted options listed for each meal.

- Where it is listed in a meal to have a tablespoon or teaspoon of extra virgin olive oil, any of the following oils may also be used instead:

  - Macadamia oil

  - Coconut oil

  - Flax-seed oil

  - Avocado oil

Acceptable Food Sources

If you are looking to substitute in alternate food sources in the meal plans, that's fine too. The following is a list of foods that provide satiety and micronutrients. I recommend using the meal plans as they are (especially to start) but the following foods are good as well. There is nothing "magic" about them, but they are good staples for any diet.

PROTEIN

- Turkey breast (skinless)

- Chicken breast (skinless)

- White fish (cod, halibut, flounder, sole, haddock, orange roughy, pickerel, trout)

- Tuna (canned in water)

- Wild salmon

- Shrimp

- Egg whites

- Inside round steak (lean)

- Flank steak (lean)

- Lean pork cuts

- Lean bison cuts

- Extra lean ground-beef

- Extra lean ground-turkey

- Extra lean ground-chicken

- Low-fat cottage cheese (1% or lower)

CARBOHYDRATES

- Any long-grain rice (brown, jasmine, wild, basmati, white)

- Large rice cakes

- Mini rice cakes

- Oatmeal (not instant)

- Cream of wheat

- Potatoes

- Sweet potatoes

- Yams

- Fruit (all types)

- Garden variety vegetables

- Cruciferous vegetables (*broccoli, cauliflower*)

- Cucumber

- Asparagus

- Squash

- Celery

- Spinach

- Kale

- Pepper

- Zucchini (etc.)

FATS

- Flax seed oil

- Macadamia oil

- Avocado oil

- Extra virgin olive oil

- Coconut oil

- Avocado

- Natural Peanut Butter

- Nuts (mixed)

- Cashews

- Hazelnuts

- Almonds

- Walnuts

- Pecan

- Macadamia

- Seeds

- Flax

- Pin

- Pumpkin

- Sunflower

Part 4.

The Complete List of Workouts & Diet Plans

the
COMPLETE HGS
LIST *of* WORKOUTS

A paperback isn't ideal for printable workout programs. To get a free, formatted, printable version of these workouts, please visit this secret link:

scottabelfitness.com/hgsworkouts

To see demonstrations of any exercise here, see my video exercise library:

scottabelfitness.com/library

Note that with this link, every video is free and open to the public... so share away.

As explained above, the workouts below are all in the format:

1a) Name of exercise   # of sets   X   # of reps

So for example "5 X 5" would mean 5 sets of 5 reps for each set.

WORKOUT 1.

Exercise	Sets X Reps
1a) DB or BB Squats	5 X 5
1b) DB Incline Press	5 X 8-10
1c) DB or BB Upright Rows	5 X 20
2a) Pull-downs Behind the Head	4 X 12-15
2b) 2 Arm DB Curls	4 X 20
3a) One-arm DB triceps extension	4 X 5-6 EA
3b) Any sit-up or leg raise variation	4 X 12-20

WORKOUT 2.

Exercise	Sets X Reps
1a) Seated cable rows	5 X 15-20
1b) Triceps Dips Between Benches	5 X 15-20
2a) Seated Cable Flyes	4 X 8-12
2b) Leg Extensions	4 X 20
3a) Seated DB Shoulder press	4 X 8-12
3b) Alternate Hammer Curls	4 X 5 EA
3c) Any sit-ups or leg raise variation	3-4 X 12-20

WORKOUT 3.

Exercise	Sets X Reps
1) Incline DB Press	5 X 5
2a) Seated Side Laterals	4 X 20
2b) Straight Arm Pull-downs	4 X 15-20
2c) One-Leg Leg Press*	4 X 20
3a) Seated Alternate DB Curls	4 X 5-6 EA
3b) Lying Triceps extensions	4 X 12-15
3c) Continue One Leg Press as directed above	

* On these types of workouts, only do ONE SIDE of a unilateral movement unless otherwise indicated. So for exercise 2c) you will do left side one leg press the first round of sequence 2 and you will do the right side on the second round of sequence 2. So, one-leg leg press will spill into exercise 3 in order to complete all four sets on each side.

WORKOUT 4.

Exercise	Sets X Reps
1a) DB Bent Lateral Raises	5 X 12-15
1b) Flat DB Flyes	5 X 8-10
1c) BW Bulgarian Split Squat*	5 X 20 EL
2a) Reverse Grip Pull-downs	4 X 8-10
2b) Continue Split Squat as above	X 20 EL
3a) One-arm DB concentration curls	4 X 8-10
3b) One-arm Reverse Grip Triceps Pushdowns	4 X 15-20

*Again this is a single side movement, so do right or left leg on the first round, then the other leg on the next round and continue till you've done all five sets for each leg.

WORKOUT 5.

Exercise	Sets X Reps
1a) Cable Crossovers	5 X 15-20
1b) One-arm DB Rows	5 X 5 EA
1c) DB Single Leg Lunges*	5 X 8-10 EL
2a) Front Alternate DB Raises	4 X 12-15
2b) Over Rope Triceps Extensions	4 X 12-15
2c) Continue left over Single Leg Lunges	till all 5 sets
3a) One-arm Zottman Curls	4 X 5 EA
3b) Any sit-up or leg raise variation	4 X 12-15

* Single leg lunge is done only one side per round –so left leg on the first round of 1c and right leg on the second round – Therefore this exercise continues into the next sequence until all five sets are complete.

WORKOUT 6.

Exercise	Sets X Reps
1a) Flat DB or BB Press	5 X 5
1b) DB Squats	5 X 5
2a) Seated DB Shoulder Press	4 X 5
2b) Alternating Pull-downs (palms face each other)	4 X 8-10
2c) Any sit-ups or leg raise variation	4 X 15-20
3a) Triceps Pushdowns	4 X 8-10
3b) Standing Simultaneous DB Curls	4 X 20

WORKOUT 7.

Exercise	Sets X Reps
1a) Cable or machine rear delts	5 X 15-20
1b) Low Incline DB Flyes	5 X 10-12
1c) DB or BB alternating lunges	5 X 5 EL
2a) One-arm DB Triceps Extension	4 X 15-20
2b) One-arm Preacher Curls	4 X 15-20
3a) One-arm Reverse Grip Pull-downs	4 X 8-10
3b) Any sit-up or leg raise variation	4 X 12-15

WORKOUT 8.

Exercise	Sets X Reps
1a) Leg Press	5 X 20
1b) 2 Arms DB Front Raises	5 X 20
1c) Lying Triceps Extensions	5 X 5
2a) One-arm Low Pulley Rows	4 X 12-15 ES
2b) Any sit-ups or leg raise variation	4 X 12-15
2c) High Incline DB Press	4 X 20
3) Standing Single Arm DB Curls	4 X 15 EA

WORKOUT 9.

Exercise	Sets X Reps
1a) DB Concentration Curls	5 X 5
1b) Cable or Tubing One-arm Triceps Kickback	5 X 20
1c) One-arm Cable Side Laterals	5 X 15 ES
2a) DB Sumo Squat	4 X 20
2b) High Angle Seated Rows	4 X 15-20
3a) Low Incline DB flyes	4 X 5
3b) Any sit-ups or leg raise variation	4 X 12-15

WORKOUT 10.

Exercise	Sets X Reps
1a) Seated Machine Chest Press	5 X 12-15
1b) DB Bent Rows	5 X 8-10
1c) Any sit-ups or leg raise variation	5 X 15-20
2a) DB or BB Shrugs	4 X 5
2b) Low Pulley Triceps Rope Extensions	4 X 12-15
2c) Single Leg Reverse Lunges *	4 X 20 EL
3a) One-arm DB Hammer Curl	4 X 5 EA

3b) Continue Single Leg Reverse Lunges till all four sets of each side are completed

* Single Side movement is done only one side per round – so right side on the first round, left side on the second round and this means this exercise will be continued into the next sequence till all four sets are complete.

WORKOUT 11.

Exercise	Sets X Reps
1a) 2 Arm Reverse Grip Triceps Pushdowns *	5 X 15-20
1b) Seated Side lateral Raise	5 X 12-15
1c) BB or Machine Preacher Curls	5 X 5
2a) Leg extension	4 X 15-20
2b) Incline DB Press	4 X 5
3a) One-arm DB rows **	4 X 5
3b) Any sit-ups or leg raise variation	4 X 15-20

* Instead of a bar or rope attachment, you will need to attach two "D"-shaped handles (single hand grip) to a single cable to do this exercise.

** Rest a bit between doing each side; remember we don't want too much oxygen debt.

WORKOUT 12.

Exercise	Sets X Reps
1a) Back Squats (*or* Front Squats *or* DB Squats)	5 X 20
1b) DB concentration Curl	5 X 10-12
2a) Reverse Grip Pull-down	4 X 12-15
2b) DB Lying Triceps Extensions with hammer grip	4 X 15-20
3a) Flat DB Press	4 X 5
3b) Cable Rear Delts (any version)	4 X 15-20
3c) Any abs crunch variation	4 X 15-20

WORKOUT 13.

Exercise	Sets X Reps
1a) Seated or Standing Alternate DB Curls	5 X 5 EA
1b) Triceps Pushdown	5 X 12-15
1c) 2-arm DB front raise	5 X 20
2a) Wide Grip Seated Row	4 X 15-20
2b) DB or BB Alternating Lunge	4 X 5 EL
3a) Low Incline DB flye	4 X 15-20
3b) Any sit-up, leg raise, or crunch variation	4 X 15-20

WORKOUT 14.

Exercise	Sets X Reps
1a) Seated Side Lateral	5 X 12-15
1b) BW Single Leg Split Bulgarian Split Squats	5 X 15-20 EL
2a) Close Grip Pull-down	4 X 15-20
2b) DB or BB Lying Triceps Extensions	4 X 5
3a) Seated Machine Cable flye	4 X 15-20
3b) Single Arm DB Preacher Curls	4 X 5 EA
3c) any crunch variation	4 X 20

WORKOUT 15.

Exercise	Sets X Reps
1a) Alternating Pull-downs (palms facing each other)	5 X 5
1b) Alternate DB Triceps Extensions (seated)	5 X 5
1c) Leg extension	5 X 15-20
2a) One-arm Cable Side Lateral Raises	4 X 15-20
2b) One-arm Zottman Curl	4 X 5
3a) Flat DB Bench Press	4 X 15-20
3b) Any leg raise, sit-up, or crunch variation	4 X 15-20

WORKOUT 16.

Exercise	Sets X Reps
1a) Low Incline DB Press	5 X 5
1b) Bent DB Lateral Raise	5 X 5
1c) DB Squats	5 X 15-20
2a) Pull-downs to the front	4 X 12-15
2b) Standing Single Arm DB curls	4 X 15-20 ES
3a) DB Triceps French Press	4 X 8-12
3b) Any sit-up (or leg raise or crunch variation)	4 X 20

WORKOUT 17.

Exercise	Sets X Reps
1a) Seated DB Shoulder Press	5 X 5
1b) Cable Crossover	5 X 15-20
1c) DB Sumo Squat	5 X 15-20
2a) One-arm DB Row	4 X 5 EA
2b) One-arm Hammer Curl	4 X 5EA
3a) Overhead Rope Triceps extensions	4 X 15-20
3b) Any crunch variation	4 X 15-20

WORKOUT 18.

Exercise	Sets X Reps
1a) BB or DB Shrug	5 X 5
1a) One-Leg Leg Press	5 X 5 EL
1c) Flat DB flyes	5 X 5
2a) Bent DB row	4 X 12-15
2b) Triceps dips between benches	4 X 15-20
3a) Alternate DB curl	4 X 12-15 ES
3b) Any sit-up, leg raise, or crunch variation	4 X 15-20

WORKOUT 19.

Exercise	Sets X Reps
1a) Single-leg leg extension	5 X 8-12
1b) DB alternate front raise	5 X 8-12 ES
2a) One-arm Preacher Curl	4 X 12-15
2b) One-arm Pushdown	4 X 15-20
3a) Cable Crossover	4 X 12-15
3b) Straight Arm Pull-down	4 X 15-20
3c) Any crunch variation	4 X 15-20

WORKOUT 20.

Exercise	Sets X Reps
1a) Triceps Pushdown	5 X 8-12
1b) Front Squats, Back Squats or DB Squats	5 X 20
1c) Seated Side Lateral	5 X 15-20
2a) Alternate DB Curl	4 X 5
2b) Close Grip Pull-down	4 X 8-12
3a) High Incline DB Press	4 X 12-15
3b) Any sit-ups, leg raise or crunch variation	4 X 15-20

WORKOUT 21.

Exercise	Sets X Reps
1a) DB Incline Press	5 X 5
1b) DB Squats	5 X 5
1c) Seated Shoulder Press	5 X 5
2a) Seated Row	4 X 15-20
2b) DB Lying triceps extensions w/ hammer grip	4 X 15-20
3a) DB concentration curl	4 X 12-15 EA
3b) Any sit-ups, leg raise or crunch variation	4 X 15-20

WORKOUT 22.

Exercise	Sets X Reps
1a) One-arm DB Row	5 X 15-20
1b) One DB triceps extension	5 X 5
2a) Flat DB Bench Press	4 X 5
2b) BW Bulgarian Split Squat*	4 X 15-20
3a) Cable Rear Delt	4 X 15-20
3b) One-arm Zottman Curl	4 X 12-15 ES

3c) Continue Bulgarian Split Squat from complex 2

* Do only one leg per round in complex 2. Therefore, you would do right leg on the first round of exercise 2b) and left leg on the second round. So to complete all four sets of Bulgarian Split Squats, this exercise will spill into complex 3.

WORKOUT 23.

Exercise	Sets X Reps
1a) One-arm Cable Bent lateral	5 X 15-20 ES
1b) One-arm DB Preacher Curl	5 X 12-15 EA
2a) Alternating Lunges BB or DB	4 X 5 EL
2b) Pull-downs to Front	4 X 12-15
3a) Flat DB flyes	4 X 15-20
3b) Cable or Tubing Triceps kickbacks	4 X 15-20
3c) Any sit-ups, leg raise or crunch variation	4 X 15-20

WORKOUT 24.

Exercise	Sets X Reps
1a) Cable Crossover	5 X 15-20
1b) Bent Rows BB or DB	5 X 5
2a) Overhead Triceps Rope Extensions	4 X 12-15
2b) DB Sumo Squat	4 X 20
2c) DB curls *or* tubing curls *or* cable simultaneous biceps curls	4 X 20 EA
3a) Seated Shoulder Press, DB *or* machine	4 X 15-20
3b) Any sit-up, crunch or leg raise variation	4 X 15-20

WORKOUT 25.

Exercise	Sets X Reps
1a) DB Lying triceps extensions with Hammer Grip	5 X 5
1b) Cable Rear Delts, any variation	5 X 15-20
1c) DB Squats	5 X 5
2a) Alternate DB Curl	4 X 12-15EA
2b) Straight Arm Pull-down	4 X 15-20
3a) High Incline DB Press	5 X 8-12
3b) Any sit-up, leg raise, or crunch variation	4 X 15-20

WORKOUT 26.

Exercise	Sets X Reps
1a) Flat DB Press	5 X 5
1b) 2 Arm DB Bent Row	5 X 12-15
1c) Seated DB Shoulder Press	5 X 5
2a) Single Leg Reverse Lunge	4 X 20 EL
2b) Single Arm Hammer Curl	4 X 5 EA
3a) Triceps Dips Between Benches *or* Dip Machine	4 X 15-20
3b) Any sit-ups, leg raise, *or* crunch variation	4 X 15-20

WORKOUT 27.

Exercise	Sets X Reps
1a) Single Arm Reverse Grip Pull-downs	5 X 5
1b) Single Arm Cable Side Laterals	5 X 15-20
2a) Triceps Pushdown	4 X 8-12
2b) 2 Arm DB Standing Curl	4 X 20
2c) Any sit-up, leg raise or crunch variation	4 X 15-20
3a) Leg extension	4 X 15-20
3b) Seated Chest Press machine	4 X 12-15

WORKOUT 28.

Exercise	Sets X Reps
1a) Close Grip Bench, elbows wide (*or* with DB)	5 X 5
1b) DB Bent lateral	5 X 15-20
1c) Leg Press	5 X 15-20
2a) Incline DB Press	4 X 8-12
2b) Seated Cable Row	4 X 20
3a) BB Curls or DB Alternate Curls	4 X 12-15 EA
3b) Any sit-up, leg raise, or crunch variation	4 X 15-20

WORKOUT 29.

Exercise	Sets X Reps
1a) Alternating Pull-downs (hands facing each other)	5 X 5
1b) BB or DB Alternating Lunge	5 X 5 EL
1c) Low Incline flye	5 X 20
2a) Seated Side Lateral Raise	4 X 15-20
2b) 2 Arm Preacher Curls, any kind	4 X 12-15
3a) Overhead Rope Triceps Extensions	4 X 15-20
3b) Any sit-ups, leg raise, or crunch variation	4 X 15-20

WORKOUT 30.

Exercise	Sets X Reps
1a) Seated DB Shoulder Press	5 X 5
1b) Low Incline DB Press	5 X 5
2a) Reverse Grip Pull-down	4 X 8-12
2b) Bulgarian Split Squat*	4 X 15-20
2c) DB Concentration Curl	4 X 8-12 EA
3a) 2 Arm DB Front Raise	4 X 15-20
3b) Continue Split Squat from above	
3c) Triceps Dips Between Benches	4 X 15-20

* Bulgarian Split Squats are done only one leg each round of the complex. So if you do right leg on the first round of the complex – you do left leg on next round. And in order to complete all four sets, this exercise will spill into sequence 3, as outlined above.

WORKOUT 31.

Exercise	Sets X Reps
1a) Bent Rows BB or DB	5 X 12-15
1b) Upright Rows BB or DB	5 X 15-20
2a) One-arm DB Preacher Curl	4 X 8-12
2b) One-arm Reverse Grip Pushdowns	4 X 12-15
2c) Single Leg Lunges *	4 X 20
3a) Seated Chest flyes machine or cables	4 X 15-20
3b) Continue Single Leg Lunges till at 4 sets complete	
3c) Any sit-ups, leg raise, or crunch variation	4 X 15-20

* Single Leg Lunges are done one leg each round in sequence 2. So, if you do left leg for set one, you will do right leg for set two. This means in order to complete all four sets this exercise will spill into exercise sequence 3 as outlined above.

WORKOUT 32.

Exercise	Sets X Reps
1a) BB or DB Shrug	5 X 5
1b) One-Leg Leg Press	5 X 5 EL
1c) One-arm Hammer Curl	5 X 5 EA
2a) Flat DB flyes	4 X 12-15
2b) Seated DB Triceps French Press	4 X 15-20
3a) Close Grip Pull-down	4 X 12-15
3b) Any sit-ups, leg raise or crunch variation	4 X 15-20

WORKOUT 33.

Exercise	Sets X Reps
1a) One-arm DB Row	5 X 12-15 ES
1b) Standing One-arm DB Curl	5 X 15-20 EA
2a) Seated Chest Press Machine	4 X 15-20
2b) Seated Side Lateral	4 X 15-20
3a) DB Alternating Lunge	4 X 12-15 EL
3b) Triceps Pushdown	4 X 15-20
3c) Any sit-up, leg raise or crunch variation	4 X 15-20

WORKOUT 34.

Exercise	Sets X Reps
1a) BB or DB Squat	5 X 5
1b) One-arm DB Triceps Extensions	5 X 5
2a) Pull-downs Behind the Head	4 X 12-15
2b) 2 Arm DB front Raise	4 X 20
3a) High Incline DB Press	4 X 8-12
3b) Alternate Hammer Curl	4 X 8-12 EA
3c) Any sit-up, leg raise, or crunch variation	4 X 15-20

WORKOUT 35.

Exercise	Sets X Reps
1a) Seated DB Shoulder Press	5 X 5
1b) One-arm Zottman Curl	5 X 5 EA
2a) Leg Press	4 X 15-20
2b) Cable Crossover	4 X 12-15
2c) Cable or Tubing Triceps Kickbacks	4 X 15-20
3a) One-arm Cable Bent Row	4 X 12-15 ES
3b) Any sit-up, leg raise or crunch variation	4 X 15-20

WORKOUT 36.

Exercise	Sets X Reps
1a) Flat DB or BB Bench Press	5 X 5
1b) Bent DB lateral	5 X 15-20
1c) BW Bulgarian Split Squat *	5 X 15-20
2a) Bent DB or BB Row	4 X 8-12
2b) Continue Bulgarian Split Squats till all 5 sets completed	
3a) Triceps Overhead Rope Extensions	4 X 8-12
3b) Standing Simultaneous DB Curls	4 X 20 EA
3c) Any sit-up, leg raise or crunch variation	4 X 15-20

* Bulgarian Split Squats are done only one leg per round. So if you do left leg on the first round of sequence 1 – you will do right leg on the second set of sequence 1. Therefore to complete all five sets for each leg, this exercise will spill into sequence 2.

WORKOUT 37.

Exercise	Sets X Reps
1a) Seated Alternate DB Curl	5 X 5EA
1b) Single Leg Lunges *	5 X 15-20
1c) Straight Arm Pull-down	5 X 15-20
2a) Triceps Dips Between Benches	4 X 15-20
2b) DB alternate Front Raise	4 X 8-12 ES
2c) Continue Single Leg Lunges till all 5 sets completed	
3a) Low Incline DB flye	4 X 15-20
3b) Any sit-up, leg raise or crunch variation	4 X 15-20

* This single leg exercise is done only one side per round. So if you do single leg lunge with right leg for the first round of sequence 1, then you would do right leg for set number two of sequence 1. Therefore this exercise will spill into exercise sequence 2 in order to complete all five required sets.

WORKOUT 38.

Exercise	Sets X Reps
1a) Leg Extensions	5 X 8-12
1b) One-arm Cable Concentration Curls	5 X 15-20 EA
1c) One-arm Cable Pushdown	5 X 15-20 EA
2a) Low Incline DB Press	4 X 12-15
2b) Alternating/Simultaneous DB Bent Rows	4 X 15-20 ES
3a) One-arm Cable Side Lateral	4 X 15-20 ES
3b) Any sit-up, leg raise, *or* crunch variation	4 X 15-20

WORKOUT 39.

Exercise	Sets X Reps
1a) Flat DB or BB Bench Press	5 X 5
1b) DB or BB Squat	5 X 5
2a) Seated DB Shoulder Press	4 X 15-20
2b) Alternate DB Curl	4 X 8-12 EA
3a) 2 Arm Reverse Grip Triceps Pushdowns *	4 X 15-20
3b) Seated Cables Rows with a rope	4 X 15-20
3c) Any sit-up, leg raise or crunch variation	4 X 15-20

* This exercise is done with single arm D-handles attached to a cable.

WORKOUT 40.

Exercise	Sets X Reps
1a) BB Cheat Curls	5 X 10-12
or Standing Alternate DB Curls	
1b) Overhead Rope Triceps Extensions	5 X 12-15
2a) Standing DB Side Lateral Raises	4 X 20
2b) Alternating DB Lunge	4 X 5EL
2c) Low Incline DB Press	4 X 8-12
3a) Leaning Cable (*or* Tubing Pull-downs/Pull ins)	4 X 15-20
3b) Any sit-up, leg raise, or crunch variation	4 X 15-20

WORKOUT 41.

Exercise	Sets X Reps
1a) One-arm DB Rows	5 X 12-15
(one side per round)	
1b) One-arm DB Front Raises	5 X 15-20
(one side per round)	
1c) One-Leg Leg Extensions	5 X 15-20
(one side per round)	
2a) Seated Chest Press	4 X 12-15
2b) Triceps Dips Between Benches	4 X 15-20
3a) One-arm High Angle Cable Curls	4 X 15-20 EA
3b) Any sit-up, leg raise, or crunch variation	4 X 15-20

* On triplex one, you would do each exercise for the right side, then do each exercise for the left side, and this would constitute one full set. And yes: you repeat until all five sets are complete. This triplex should not require any rest when going from one side to the next, or from set to set.

WORKOUT 42.

Exercise	Sets X Reps
1a) DB or BB Squat	5 X 5
1b) DB Concentration Curl	5 X 5 EA
1c) One-arm Triceps Pushdown	5 X 15-20 EA
2a) Seated DB Shoulder Press	4 X 15-20
2b) Low Incline DB Flye	4 X 8-12
3a) Seated Cable Row	4 X 15-20
3b) Any sit-up, leg raise, or crunch variation	4 X 15-20

WORKOUT 43.

Exercise	Sets X Reps
1a) One-arm Low Cable Rows, standing	5 X 8-12
1b) One-arm DB triceps extension, seated	5 X 5
2a) One-Leg Leg Press	4 X 5 EL
2b) Cable Crossover	4 X 15-20
3a) 2-arm preacher curls, machine optional	4 X 12-15
3b) DB or BB upright row	4 X 15-20
3c) Any sit-up, leg raise, or crunch variation	4 X 15-20

WORKOUT 44.

Exercise	Sets X Reps
1a) Alternating Pull-downs with palms facing each other	5 X 5 ES
1b) Standing DB Side Lateral Raises	5 X 15-20
1c) Seated Alternate DB Triceps Extensions	5 X 5 EA
2a) Seated Chest Flye	4 X 15-20
2b) Single Leg Lunge (not alternating) BB *or* DB	4 X 5 EL
3a) Alternate Hammer Curl	4 X 8-12
3b) Any sit-up, leg raise, or crunch variation	4 X 15-20

WORKOUT 45.

Exercise	Sets X Reps
1a) Leg Extension	5 X 15-20
1b) Flat DB Press, feet up on bench	5 X 5
1c) 2-arm DB front raise	5 X 20
2a) Bent Over DB or BB row	4 X 15-20
2b) Triceps Dips Between Benches *or* Bar Dips	4 X 15-20
3a) One-arm DB Preacher Curl	4 X 8-12 EA
3b) Any sit-ups, leg raise, *or* crunch variation	4 X 15-20

WORKOUT 46.

Exercise	Sets X Reps
1a) Seated DB Shoulder Press	5 X 5
1b) Leg Press	5 X 15-20
2a) Low Incline DB Press	4 X 12-15
2b) Reverse Grip Pull-down	4 X 12-15
3a) Triceps Pushdown	4 X 8-12
3b) BB Curls *or* Cable 2 Arm Curls	4 X 15-20
3c) Any Sit-up, leg raise, *or* crunch variation	4 X 15-20

WORKOUT 47.

Exercise	Sets X Reps
1a) One-arm Cable Side Laterals *	5 X 15-20
(one side per round)	
1b) One-arm DB Rows	5 X 5
(one side per round)	
1c) One-arm Zottman Curls	5 X 5
(one side per round)	
2a) Flat DB Flyes, feet up on bench	4 X 12-15
2b) DB Sumo Squat	4 X 20
3a) BB or DB Triceps Close Grip Bench Press	4 X 15-20
3b) Any sit-up, leg raise, or crunch variation	4 X 15-20

* On triplex one, you would do each exercise for the right side, then do each exercise for the left side, and this would constitute one full set. And yes: you repeat until all five sets are complete. This triplex should not require any rest when going from one side to the next, or from set to set.

WORKOUT 47.

Exercise	Sets X Reps
1a) Incline DB or BB Press	5 X 5
1b) DB Bent Lateral	5 X 15-20
2a) One-Leg Leg Press * (one side per round)	4 X 20
2b) Reverse Grip One-arm Pull-down (one side per round)	4 X 12-15
2c) One-arm DB Preacher Curls (one side per round)	4 X 15-20
3a) Lying DB or BB Triceps Extensions	4 X 20
3b) Any sit-up, leg raise, *or* crunch variation	4 X 15-20

* On triplex two, you would do each exercise for the right side, then do each exercise for the left side, and this would constitute one full set. And yes: you repeat until all five sets are complete. This triplex should not require any rest when going from one side to the next, or from set to set.

WORKOUT 47.

Exercise	Sets X Reps
1a) Seated DB or Machine Shoulder Press	5 X 20
1b) Cable Crossover	5 X 20
2a) Seated Alternate DB Curl	4 X 5 EA
2b) Overhead Rope Extensions	4 X 15-20
2c) BW Bulgarian Split Squats *	4 X 15-20
3a) High to Low Angle Seated One-arm Pulldowns / Rows	4 X 12-15 ES
3b) Continue Split Squats till all sets complete	
3c) Any sit-up, leg raise, or crunch variation	4 X 15-20

* On exercise 2c, you only do one side per round. So if you do left leg for the first round in sequence 2c), then you would do right leg for the second round of sequence 2c). Therefore to complete all sets, this exercise will continue into exercise sequence 3.

WORKOUT 50.

Exercise	Sets X Reps
1a) One-arm DB Row	5 X 5 EA
1b) One-arm Cable Bent Laterals	5 X 15-20 EA
2a) Flat Flys or Machine Fly	4 X 12-15
2b) Leg Extension	4 X 8-12
3a) Triceps Pushdown	4 X 12-15
3b) 2 arm Preacher Curl	4 X 12-15
3c) Any sit-up, leg raise, *or* crunch variation	4 X 15-20

WORKOUT 51.

Exercise	Sets X Reps
1a) Flat BB or DB Press	5 X 12-15
feet up on end of bench, if possible	
1b) Alternate DB front raise	5 X 12-15
1c) One-arm Hammer Curl	5 X 5 EA
2a) Reverse Grip Pull-down	4 X 12-15
2b) Lying Triceps Extensions, DB or BB	4 X 12-15
3a) BB *or* DB Squat	4 X 20
3b) Any sit-up, leg raise *or* crunch variation	4 X 15-20

WORKOUT 52.

Exercise	Sets X Reps
1a) BW Chins or Pull-downs to Front	5 X 12-15
1b) Alternating BB or DB lunge	5 X 20 EL
2a) Low Incline Fly	4 X 8-12
2b) Rear Delts Machine or Cable Rear Delts	4 X 15-20
3a) One-arm DB Triceps Extensions	4 X 15-20
3b) One-arm DB Concentration Curls	4 X 15-20
3c) Any sit-up, leg raise or crunch variation	4 X 15-20

WORKOUT 53.

Exercise	Sets X Reps
1a) Low Incline BB *or* DB Press	5 X 5
1b) Leg Press	5 X 15-20
2a) One-arm DB Row (one side per round)	4 X 15-20
2b) One-arm Standing DB Curl (one side per round)	4 X 20
2c) One-arm Triceps Pushdowns (one side per round)	4 X 12-15
3a) Seated DB or Machine Shoulder Press	4 X 15-20
3b) Any sit-up, leg raise or crunch variation	4 X 15-20

* On exercise sequence 2, you will do all three exercises on one side, then do all three exercises on the other side, and this constitutes one set. Continue one side at a time till all four sets are completed. There should be no need to rest between each side.

WORKOUT 54.

Exercise	Sets X Reps
1a) One-Leg Leg Press	5 X 5 EL
1b) One-arm DB Shrug	5 X 5 ES
(DB in front, not at the side)	
1b) One-arm Reverse Grip Triceps Pushdowns	5 X 20 EA
2a) Seated Cable Row	4 X 12-15
2b) BB Cheat Curls or Seated Alternate Curls	4 X 15-20
3a) Seated Chest Press Machine	4 X 20
3b) Any sit-up, leg raise, *or* crunch variation	4 X 15-20

WORKOUT 55.

Exercise	Sets X Reps
1a) DB Squats	5 X 20
1b) Bent DB Lateral	5 X 15-20
1c) Seated Machine or Cable Flyes	5 X 15-20
2a) High Angle Cable Biceps Curls	4 X 15-20
2b) Short ROM MB Diamond Push-ups for Triceps	4 X 12-15
3a) Straight Arm Pull-down	4 X 15-20
3b) Any sit-up, leg raise, or crunch variation	4 X 15-20

WORKOUT 56.

Exercise	Sets X Reps
1a) Alternating Cable Pull-downs	5 X 5 ES
(use palms facing each other)	
1b) DB Flat Bench Press	5 X 12-15
2a) Seated DB Shoulder Press	4 X 12-15
2b) DB Alternating Lunge	4 X 20 EL
3a) DB Triceps French Press	4 X 20
3b) DB Alternate Hammer Curl	4 X 5 EA
3c) Any sit-up, leg raise, *or* crunch variation	4 X 15-20

WORKOUT 57.

Exercise	Sets X Reps
1a) Leg Extension	5 X 15-20
1b) Seated Cable Row	5 X 12-15
2a) Low Incline DB flye	4 X 8-12
2b) 2 Arm DB Front Raise	4 X 20
2c) Any sit-up, leg raise, *or* crunch variation	4 X 15-20
3a) One-arm Hammer Curl	4 X 5 EA
3b) Seated One-arm DB Triceps Extension	4 X 5 EA

WORKOUT 58.

Exercise	Sets X Reps
1a) Seated DB Side Lateral	5 X 12-15
1b) DB or BB Bent Over Row	5 X 5
1c) Overhead Rope Triceps Extensions	5 X 15-20
2a) Concentration DB Curl	4 X 12-15
2b) Bulgarian Split Squat, one side per round	4 X 15-20
3a) Seated Machine Chest Press	4 X 15-20
3b) Continue Bulgarian Split Squat	
3c) Any sit-up, leg raise, *or* crunch variation	4 X 15-20

* Bulgarian Split Squats are done only one side per round in sequence 2. This means if you do left leg on the first set through, you will do right leg on the second set through. Therefore, Bulgarian Split Squats will continue into sequence 3 until all four sets are complete.

WORKOUT 59.

Exercise	Sets X Reps
1a) DB or BB Incline Press	5 X 5
1b) Single-Leg Leg Extensions	5 X 12-15 EL
2a) Alternating Front DB Raises	4 X 5 EA
2b) Straight Arm Pull-downs	4 X 20
3a) Lying Triceps Extensions DB or BB	4 X 15-20
3b) Machine Preacher Curls	4 X 15-20
3c) Any sit-up, leg raise, *or* crunch variation	4 X 15-20

WORKOUT 60.

Exercise	Sets X Reps
1a) One-arm DB Shoulder Press	5 X 5 EA
1b) One-arm DB preacher curl	5 X 5 EA
2a) One-arm triceps pushdown	4 X 12-15
2b) Leg Press	4 X 15-20
3a) Flat DB flys	4 X 20
3b) Seated Cable rows, high to low angle	4 X 12-15
3c) Any sit-up, leg raise, *or* crunch variation	4 X 15-20

WORKOUT 61.

Exercise	Sets X Reps
1a) Incline DB flys	5 X 12-15
1b) DB squats	5 X 15-20
2a) DB seated side lateral	4 X 8-12
2b) Wide-grip pull-down	4 X 12-15
2c) DB concentration curls *	4 X 15-20EA
3a) One-arm Overhead Triceps Rope Extensions	4 X 12-15 EA
3b) Any sit-up, leg raise, *or* crunch variation	4 X 15-20

WORKOUT 62.

Exercise	Sets X Reps
1a) DB *or* BB Squat	5 X 5
1b) Machine shoulder press	5 X 8-12
1c) Standing BB curl	5 X 15-20
2a) Close-grip pull-down	4 X 12-15
2b) Close-grip bench press (elbows flared)	4 X 15-20
3a) Seated cable fly	4 X 20
3b) Any sit-up, leg raise, *or* crunch variation	4 X 15-20

WORKOUT 63.

Exercise	Sets X Reps
1a) Bent rows	5 X 8-12
1b) Alternate front DB raises	5 X 12-15
2a) Incline machine chest press	4 X 15-20
2b) Rope triceps pushdown	4 X 12-15
2c) Single-leg leg press *	4 X 15
3a) Continue single leg press until all sets complete	
3b) Any sit-up, leg raise, or crunch variation	4 X 15-20

* Single-Leg Leg Press is done only one side per round in sequence 2. This means if you do left leg on the first set through, you will do right leg on the second set through. Therefore, Single-Leg Leg Press will continue into sequence 3a until all four sets are complete.

WORKOUT 64.

Exercise	Sets X Reps
1a) Triceps pushdown	5 X 5
1b) One-arm Zottman curl	5 X 12-15 EA
2a) BB flat bench press, feet up on bench	4 X 12-15
2b) Supported Seated row	4 X 15-20
3a) Squats Smith machine *	4 X 12-15
3b) DB Upright Row	4 X 15-20
3b) Any sit-up, leg raise, *or* crunch variation	4 X 15-20

* Feet together and far forward; the goal is to target your glutes.

WORKOUT 65.

Exercise	Sets X Reps
1a) Leg press	5 X 20
1b) Chest fly machine	5 X 15-20
1c) Incline diamond push-ups* (triceps)	5 X 8-12
2a) One-arm DB row	4 X 12-15 ES
2b) One-arm DB shoulder press	4 X 15 ES
3a) One-arm hammer curl	4 X 15-20 EA
3b) Any sit-up, leg raise, or crunch variation	4 X 15-20

* Pushing upper body off a bench or similar height platform with feet on the ground to create an incline plane. Can shorten ROM to complete required reps.

WORKOUT 66.

Exercise	Sets X Reps
1a) Weighted or BW dips (lean forward-chest)	5 X 8-12
1b) BB squats or Hack Squats Machine	5 X 12-15
2a) Seated Incline DB alternating bicep curls	4 X 5 EA
2b) One-arm cable row	4 X 15-20 ES
3a) Seated one-arm DB triceps extensions	4 X 15-20 EA
3b) One-arm Cable rear delt	4 X 12-15 ES
3c) Any sit-up, leg raise, *or* crunch variation	4 X 15-20

WORKOUT 67.

Exercise	Sets X Reps
1a) Reverse grip pull-down	5 X 15-20
1b) Standing one-arm DB shoulder press	5 X 8-12 ES
1c) DB Sumo Squat	5 X 20
2a) Cable cross-over	4 X 15-20
2b) Lying DB *or* BB triceps extensions	4 X 12-15
3a) Machine *or* BB Preacher Curls	4 X 15-20
3b) Any sit-up, leg raise, *or* crunch variation	4 X 15-20

WORKOUT 68.

Exercise	Sets X Reps
1a) Triceps pushdown	5 X 5
1b) DB Walking lunge	5 X 15-20 EL
2a) Standing one-arm side laterals (Cable or DB)	4 X 8-12 ES
2b) 1-Arm Cable Concentration Curls	4 X 15-20EA
3a) Machine chest press (any kind)	4 X 15-20
3b) Straight Arm Pull-down	4 X 15-20
3c) Any sit-up, leg raise, or crunch variation	4 X 15-20

WORKOUT 69.

Exercise	Sets X Reps
1a) Alternating one-arm pull-downs (palms facing each other)	5 X 20 ES
1b) Upright DB *or* BB rows	5 X 12-15
1c) Incline DB flye	5 X 15-20
2a) Standing DB bicep curl	4 X 15-20
2b) DB Reverse lunge	4 X 12-15 EL
3a) Overhead rope triceps extensions	4 X 15-20
3b) Any sit-up, leg raise, *or* crunch variation	4 X 15-20

WORKOUT 70.

Exercise	Sets X Reps
1a) DB or BB flat bench press	5 X 5
1b) Tubing *or* cable bicep curl	5 X 12-15
2a) Simultaneous DB seated shoulder press	4 X 12-15 ES
2b) DB alternating bent row	4 X 15-20 ES
3a) Alternating cable front raise	4 X 12-15 ES
3b) One-arm pushdown	4 X 15-20 EA
3c) DB or BB or smith machine squat	4 X 15-20

WORKOUT 71.

Exercise	Sets X Reps
1a) Flat DB Bench press	5 X 8-12
1b) Two-arm DB or BB front raises	5 X 20
2a) Single leg lunges DB *or* BB	4 X 15-20 EL
2b) Alternating One-arm hammer curls	4 X 5EA
2c) Wide grip seated cable row	4 X 15-20
3a) Triceps DB French Press	4 X 12-15
3b) Any crunch *or* core exercise	4 X 15-20

WORKOUT 72.

Exercise	Sets X Reps
1a) Machine Should Press (any kind)	5 X 8-12
1b) BB *or* DB Alternating Lunge	5 X 12-15 EL
1c) Triceps Bench Dip	5 X 15-20
2a) One-arm rows DB	4 X 5 ES
2b) One-arm DB Concentration Curls	4 X 5 EA
3a) Flat DB Flys	4 X 15-20
3b) Any sit-up, leg raise, *or* crunch variation	4 X 15-20

WORKOUT 73.

Exercise	Sets X Reps
1a) Standing BB biceps cheat curls	5 X 15-20
1b) DB alternating lunge	5 X 5 ES
1c) DB One-arm Side Lateral	5 X 8-12 ES
2a) DB or BB incline bench press	4 X 8-12
2b) One-arm Bent Cable	4 X 15-20 EA
or Tubing Triceps Kickbacks	
3a) Alternating seated cable row	4 X 12-15 ES
3b) Any sit-up, leg raise, *or* crunch variation	4 X 15-20

WORKOUT 74.

Exercise	Sets X Reps
1a) Seated Chest Press Machine (any kind)	5 X 12-15
1b) Rear delts machine	5 X 15-20
2a) MB Diamond Push-ups (Elbows flared, full lockout each rep)	4 X 8-12
2b) DB concentration curl	4 X 15-20 EA
2c) Bulgarian split squats *	4 X 15-20
3a) Continued Bulgarian split squat s**	
3b) Any sit-up, leg raise, or crunch variation	4 X 15-20

* MB Diamond Push-ups can be done with less ROM in order to complete the required reps

** Bulgarian Split Squats are done only one side per round in sequence 2. This means if you do left leg on the first set through, you will do right leg on the second set through. Therefore, Bulgarian Split Squats will continue into sequence 3 until all four sets are complete.

WORKOUT 75.

Exercise	Sets X Reps
1a) Leg extension	5 X 8-12
1b) Bent laterals	5 X 15
2a) One-arm row (one side per round)	4 X 5
2b) One-arm Triceps Pushdowns (one side per round)	4 X 15-20
2a) One-arm standing DB curl (one side per round)	4 X 15-20
3b) Cable Crossover	4 X 15-20
3c) Any sit-up, leg raise, *or* crunch variation	4 X 15-20

* On exercise sequence 2, you will do all three exercises on one side, then do all three exercises on the other side, and this constitutes one set. Continue one side at a time till all four sets are completed. There should be no need to rest between each side.

WORKOUT 76.

Exercise	Sets X Reps
1a) DB Flat Press	5 X 5
1b) DB Squats	5 X 5
1c) One-arm Seated Shoulder Press	5 X 5 ES
2a) Low Pulley Rope Triceps Extensions	4 X 20
2b) Close Grip Pull-down	4 X 15-20
3a) Cable concentration curl	4 X 12-15 EA
3b) Any Sit-ups, leg raise *or* crunch variation	4 X 15-20

WORKOUT 77.

Exercise	Sets X Reps
1a) Alternating Seated DB curl	5 X 5 ES
1b) DB Seated Side Lateral	5 X 12-15
2a) BW Bulgarian Split squat	4 X 20 EL
2b) Triceps Dips, regular dip bar	4 X 15-20
2c) Bent DB row	4 X 5
3a) Incline smith machine *or* any incline machine press	4 X 15-20
3b) Any sit-up, leg raise, *or* crunch variation	4 X 15-20

WORKOUT 78.

Exercise	Sets X Reps
1a) Leg Press	5 X 12-15
1b) Seated Alt DB Shoulder Press (use Hammer Grip)	5 X 8-12 ES
2a) Triceps Pushdown	4 X 15-20
2b) Two-arm preacher curls (any kind)	4 X 12-15
2c) Close Grip Pull-down	4 X 12-15
3a) Seated Machine Chest Fly	4 X 20
3b) Any sit-up, leg raise, *or* crunch variation	4 X 15-20

WORKOUT 79.

Exercise	Sets X Reps
1a) DB *or* BB upright row	5 X 12-15
1b) Leg Extension	5 X 20
2a) Wide-Grip Pulldowns (behind head)	4 X 15-20
2b) DB *or* BB Lying Triceps Extensions	4 X 5
3a) Single Arm DB Preacher Curls	4 X 5 EA
3b) Low Incline DB Flys	4 X 5
3c) Any sit-up, leg raise, *or* crunch variation	4 X 20

WORKOUT 80.

Exercise	Sets X Reps
1a) DB *or* BB Squat	5 X 5
1b) Arm Triceps Pushdown	5 X 15-20 EA
1c) DB One-arm Concentration Curls	5 X 15-20 EA
2a) 2 Arm DB Front Raise	4 X 15-20
2b) Cable *or* Machine Incline Chest Press	4 X 8-12
3a) Seated Cable Rows, low to high angle	4 X 15-20
3b) Any sit-up, leg raise, *or* crunch variation	4 X 15-20

the
COMPLETE HGS
LIST *of* MEAL PLANS

~1,200 **CALORIE** MEAL PLAN

Meal 1

- One round tablespoon of natural peanut butter and 1/2 cup of oats, **Or**

- 2 whole eggs and 35 g of dry cream of wheat, **Or**

- 1 cup of egg-whites (~250 ml) and 35 g of dry cream-of-wheat

Meal 2

- 1 can of tuna packed in water and ½ a cup of long-grain brown rice and a small salad with a teaspoon of extra virgin olive oil on top, **Or**

- 1 scoop of protein powder and 4 large rice cakes (preferable the first or third option,) **Or**

- 20 g (0.7 oz.) of nuts (about what fits in the small palm of your hand) and 4 large rice cakes

Meal 3

- 100 g (3.5 oz.) white fish and a 2 pieces of fruit, **Or**

- One scoop of protein powder and 2 pieces of fruit (berries - either frozen or fresh are a great choice and 1 cup would serve as 1 to 2 pieces of fruit)

Meal 4

- 100 g (3.5 oz.) skinless chicken or turkey breast and 100 g (3.5 oz.) of potatoes or sweet potatoes and a small salad and a teaspoon of extra virgin olive oil on top, **Or**

- 100 g (3.5 oz.) white fish (refer to 'food-sources' guide for white-fish types) with 100 g - (3.5 oz.) of potatoes or sweet potatoes and ½ a cup of brown rice and a small salad and a teaspoon of extra virgin olive oil as dressing

Meal 5

- 1 cup of low-fat cottage cheese and 1/2 a cup of oats, **Or**

- 1 cup (~250 ml) of egg-whites and a couple of pieces of fruit, **Or**

- 1 cup (~250 ml) of egg-whites and 35 g of dry cream-of-wheat

Once per week use 100 g (3.5 oz.) of lean steak as a protein source. Keep the rest of the meal the same

Once per week use 100 g wild salmon as a protein source. Keep the rest of the meal the same

Once per week have a large salad as a meal – lots of leafy greens, tablespoon of cranberries, teaspoon of seeds, palm full of crumbled walnuts, 2 to 3 tablespoons of chickpeas.

~1,500 CALORIE MEAL PLAN

Meal 1

- 1 cup of egg-whites (~250 ml) and 1/3 of a cup of dry cream-of-wheat, **Or**

- 2 whole eggs and 1/3 of a cup of dry cream of wheat, **Or**

- Two tablespoons of natural peanut butter and a 1/2 cup of oats

Meal 2

- 20 to 30 g (0.7 oz.) of nuts (about what fits in the small palm of your hand) and 5 large rice cakes, **Or**

- 1 can of tuna packed in water and ½ a cup of cooked long-grain brown rice and a small salad with a teaspoon of extra virgin olive oil on top, **Or**

- 1 scoop of protein powder and 6 large rice cakes (preferably the first or second option)

Meal 3

- 100 g (3.5 oz.) white fish and a 2 to 3 pieces of fruit, Or

- One scoop of protein powder and 2 to 3 pieces of fruit (berries - either frozen or fresh are a great choice and 1 cup would serve as 1 to 2 pieces of fruit)

- 150 g shrimp drained, ½ cup of cooked brown rice and a small salad

Meal 4

- 100 g (3.5 oz.) skinless chicken or turkey breast and 100 g (3.5 oz.) of potatoes or sweet potatoes and a small salad and a tablespoon of extra virgin olive oil on top, **Or**

- 100 g (3.5 oz.) of white fish (refer to 'food-sources' guide for white-fish types) with 100 g (3.5 oz.) of potatoes or sweet potatoes and a small salad and a tablespoon of extra virgin olive oil as dressing, **Or**

- 100 g (3.5 oz.) skinless chicken or turkey breast and ½ a cup of cooked brown rice and a small and a tablespoon of extra virgin olive oil as dressing

Meal 5

- 1 cup (~250 ml) of egg-whites and a few pieces of fruit, **Or**

- 1 cup of low-fat cottage cheese and 3/4 of a cup of oats, **Or**

- 1 cup (~250 ml) of egg-whites and a 1/3 of a cup of dry cream-of-wheat

Once per week use 100 g (3.5 oz.) of lean steak as a protein source. Keep the rest of the meal the same

Once per week use 100 g wild salmon as a protein source. Keep the rest of the meal the same

Once per week have a large salad as a meal – lots of leafy greens, tablespoon of cranberries, teaspoon of seeds, palm-full of crumbled walnuts, 2 to 3 tablespoons of chickpeas.

~1,800 **CALORIE** MEAL PLAN

Meal 1

- ½ cup of egg-whites (~125 ml), 1/3 of a cup of dry cream-of-wheat and a tablespoon of natural peanut butter, **Or**

- 3 whole eggs and a 1/3 of a cup of dry cream of wheat, **Or**

- Two tablespoons of natural peanut butter and ½ a cup of oats

Meal 2

- 20 to 30g (0.7 oz.) of nuts (about what fits in the small palm of your hand) and 5 large rice cakes, **Or**

- 1 can of tuna packed in water and 1 cup of cooked long-grain brown rice and a small salad with a teaspoon of extra virgin olive oil on top, **Or**

- 1 scoop of protein powder and 6 large rice cakes (preferably the first or second option)

Meal 3

- 120g (4.2 oz.) white fish and 3 pieces of fruit, **Or**

- One scoop of protein powder and 3 pieces of fruit (berries - either frozen or fresh are a great choice and 1 cup would serve as 1 to 2 pieces of fruit,) **Or**

- 150g shrimp drained, 1 cup of cooked brown rice and a small salad

Meal 4

- 100g (3.5 oz.) skinless chicken or turkey breast and 150 g (5.3 oz.) of potatoes or sweet potatoes and a small salad and a teaspoon of extra virgin olive oil on top, **Or**

- 100g (3.5 oz.) of white fish (refer to 'food-sources' guide for white-fish types) with 150 g (5.3 oz.) of potatoes or sweet potatoes and a small salad and a tablespoon of extra virgin olive oil as dressing, **Or**

- 100g (3.5 oz.) skinless chicken or turkey breast and 1 cup of cooked brown rice and a small salad and a teaspoon of extra virgin olive oil as dressing

Meal 5

- 1.5 cups (~250 ml) of egg-whites and a few pieces of fruit, **Or**

- 1.5 cups of low-fat cottage cheese and ¾ of a cup of oats, **Or**

- 1.5 cups (~250 ml) of egg-whites and a 1/3 of a cup of dry cream-of-wheat

Once per week sub in 100 g of lean-cut steak as a protein source in place of any of the protein sources for meal 4. Keep the rest of the meal the same.

Once per week sub in 100 g of wild salmon as a protein source in place of any of the protein sources for meal 4. Keep the rest of the meal the same.

Once per week have a large salad as a meal – lots of leafy greens, tablespoon of cranberries, teaspoon of seeds, palm-full of crumbled walnuts, 2 to 3 tablespoons of chickpeas.

~2,100 **CALORIE** MEAL PLAN

Meal 1

- Two level tablespoons of natural peanut butter and ¾ of a cup of oats, **Or**

- 3 whole eggs, 3 egg-whites and a 1/3 of a cup of dry cream of wheat, **Or**

- 1 cup of egg-whites (~250 ml), a 1/3 of a cup of dry cream-of-wheat and a level tablespoon of natural peanut butter

Meal 2

- 1.5 scoops of protein powder and 6 large rice cakes (preferably the second or third option,) **Or**

- 1 can of tuna packed in water and 1 cup of cooked long-grain brown rice and a small salad with a teaspoon of extra virgin olive oil on top, **Or**

- 20 to 30 g (0.7 oz.) of nuts (about what fits in the small palm of your hand) and 6 large rice cakes

Meal 3

- 150 g (5.3 oz.) white fish (see 'food-source' guide for selection of white-fish) and a 3 to 4 pieces of fruit, **Or**

- 150 g (5.3 oz.) lean-cut meat (see 'food-source' guide) or turkey breast and 150 g (5.3 oz.) of potatoes or sweet potatoes and a small salad and a teaspoon of extra virgin olive oil on top, **Or**

- 150 g shrimp drained, 1 cup of cooked brown rice and a small salad and a teaspoon of extra virgin olive oil

Meal 4

- 150 g (5.3 oz.) skinless chicken or turkey breast and 1 cup of cooked brown rice and a small salad and a teaspoon of extra virgin olive oil as dressing, **Or**

- 1.5 scoops of protein powder and 3 to 4 pieces of fruit (berries - either frozen or fresh are a great choice and 1 cup would serve as 1 to 2 pieces of fruit,) **Or**

- 150 g (5.3 oz.) of white fish (refer to 'food-sources' guide for white-fish types) with 150 g (5.3 oz.) of potatoes or sweet potatoes and a small salad and a tablespoon of extra virgin olive oil as dressing

Meal 5

- 1.5 cups (~250 ml) of egg-whites and 3 to 4 pieces of fruit, **Or**

- 1.5 cups of low-fat cottage cheese and ¾ of a cup of oats and a teaspoon of natural peanut butter, **Or**

- 1.5 cups (~250 ml) of egg-whites and 75 g of dry cream-of-wheat

Once per week sub in 100 g of lean-cut steak as a protein source in place of any of the protein sources for meal 4. Keep the rest of the meal the same.

Once per week sub in 100 g of wild salmon as a protein source in place of any of the protein sources for meal 4. Keep the rest of the meal the same.

Once per week have a large salad as a meal – lots of leafy greens, tablespoon of cranberries, 1 teaspoon of seeds, palm-full of crumbled walnuts, 2 to 3 tablespoons of chickpeas.

~2,400 CALORIE MEAL PLAN

Meal 1

- 1 cup of egg-whites (~250 ml), 1/3 of a cup of dry cream-of-wheat and a level tablespoon of natural peanut butter, **Or**

- Two level tablespoons of natural peanut butter and ¾ of a cup of oats, **Or**

- 3 whole eggs, 3 egg-whites and 1/3 of a cup of dry cream of wheat

Meal 2

- 20 to 30 g (0.7 oz.) of nuts (about what fits in the small palm of your hand) and 6 large rice cakes **Or**

- 1 can of tuna packed in water and 1 cup of cooked long-grain brown rice and a small salad with a teaspoon of extra virgin olive oil on top, **Or**

- 1.5 scoops of protein powder and 6 large rice cakes (preferably the first <u>or</u> second option)

Meal 3

- 200 g shrimp drained, 1 cup of cooked brown rice and a small salad, **Or**

- 150 g (5.3 oz.) white fish (see 'food-source' guide) and a 3 to 4 pieces of fruit, **Or**

- 150 g (5.3 oz.) lean- cut meat (see 'food-source' guide for allowed selection) or turkey breast and 150 g (5.3 oz.) of potatoes or sweet potatoes and a small salad and a teaspoon of extra virgin olive oil on top

Meal 4

- 150 g of white fish (refer to food sources guide for selection) and 150 g (5.3 oz.) potatoes or sweet potatoes, **Or**

- 1 cup of low-fat cottage cheese and 6 large rice cakes, **Or**

- 1 to 2 level tablespoons of natural peanut butter and 4 large rice cakes

Meal 5

- 150 g (5.3 oz.) skinless chicken or turkey breast and 1 cup of cooked brown rice and a small salad and a teaspoon of extra virgin olive oil as dressing, **Or**

- 1.5 scoops of protein powder and 3 to 4 pieces of fruit (berries - either frozen or fresh are a great choice and 1 cup would serve as 1 to 2 pieces of fruit) **Or**

- 150 g (5.3 oz.) of white fish (refer to 'food-sources' guide for selection) with 150 g (5.3 oz.) of potatoes or sweet potatoes and a small salad and a tablespoon of extra virgin olive oil as dressing

Meal 6

- 1.5 cups (~250 ml) of egg-whites and 75 g of dry cream-of-wheat **Or**

- 1.5 cups of low-fat cottage cheese and ¾ of a cup of oats **Or**

- 1.5 cups (~250 ml) of egg-whites and 3 to 4 pieces of fruit

  ○ Once per week sub in 150 g (7 oz.) of lean-cut steak as a protein source in place of any of the protein sources for meal 5. Keep the rest of the meal the same.

  ○ Once per week, sub in 150 g (7 oz.) of wild salmon as a protein source, in place of any of the protein sources for meal 5. Keep the rest of the meal the same.

~2,700 **CALORIE** MEAL PLAN

Meal 1

- 1.5 cup of egg-whites (~375 ml), 75 g of dry cream-of-wheat, **Or**

- 2 whole eggs, 4 egg-whites and 75 g of dry cream of wheat, **Or**

- 2 level tablespoons of natural peanut butter and ¾ of a cup of oats

Meal 2

- 25 to 30 g (0.7 oz.) of nuts (about what fits in the small palm of your hand) and 8 large rice cakes **Or**

- 1 can of tuna packed in water and 1 cup of cooked long-grain brown rice and a small salad with a tablespoon of extra virgin olive oil on top, **Or**

- 1.5 scoops of protein powder and 8 large rice cakes (preferably the first or second option)

Meal 3

- 200 g shrimp drained, 1 cup of cooked brown rice and a small salad and a teaspoon of extra virgin olive oil, **Or**

- 150 g (5.3 oz.) lean-cut meat (see 'food-source' guide for allowed selection) or turkey breast and 200 g (7 oz.) of potatoes or sweet potatoes and a small salad and a teaspoon of extra virgin olive oil on top, **Or**

- 200 g (7 oz.) white fish (see 'food-source' guide for selection) and a 3 to 4 pieces of fruit

Meal 4

- 2 level tablespoons of natural peanut butter and 7 large rice cakes, **Or**

- 200 g (7 oz.) of white fish (refer to food sources guide for selection) and 200 g (7 oz.) potatoes or sweet potatoes, **Or**

- 2 cups of low-fat cottage cheese and 8 large rice cakes, **Or**

- 200 g (7 oz.) of white fish (refer to food sources guide for selection) and 1 cup of cooked brown rice

Meal 5

- 150 g (5.3 oz.) skinless chicken or turkey breast and 1 cup of cooked brown rice and a small salad and a tablespoon of extra virgin olive oil as dressing, **Or**

- 2 scoops of protein powder and 3 to 4 pieces of fruit (berries - either frozen or fresh are a great choice and 1 cup would serve as 1 to 2 pieces of fruit,) **Or**

- 150 g (5.3 oz.) of white fish (refer to 'food-sources' guide for selection) with 150 g (5.3 oz.) of potatoes or sweet potatoes and a small salad and a tablespoon of extra virgin olive oil as dressing

Meal 6

- 1.5 cups (~250 ml) of egg-whites and 75 g of dry cream-of-wheat, **Or**

- 1.5 cups of low-fat cottage cheese and 1 cup of oats, Or

- 2 cups (~375 ml) of egg-whites and 3 to 4 pieces of fruit, **Or**

- 2 tablespoons of natural peanut butter and 6 to 7 large rice cakes

Once per week sub in 150 g (7 oz.) of lean-cut steak as a protein source in place of any of the protein sources for meal 5. Keep the rest of the meal the same.

Once per week sub in 150 g (7 oz.) of wild salmon as a protein source in place of any of the protein sources for meal 5. Keep the rest of the meal the same.

~3,000 **CALORIE** MEAL PLAN

Meal 1

- 2 cups of egg-whites (~500 ml), 75 g of dry cream-of-wheat, **Or**

- 3 whole eggs, 4 egg-whites and 75 g of dry cream of wheat, **Or**

- Two level tablespoons of natural peanut butter and 1 cup of oats

Meal 2

- 25 to 30 g (0.7 oz.) of nuts (about what fits in the small palm of your hand) and 10 large rice cakes, **Or**

- 1 can of tuna packed in water and 1 cups of cooked long-grain brown rice and a small salad with a 1 to 2 tablespoons of extra virgin olive oil on top, **Or**

- 1.5 scoops of protein powder and 10 large rice cakes (preferably the first <u>or</u> second option)

Meal 3

- 200 g (7 oz.) shrimp drained, 1.5 cups of cooked brown rice and a small salad and a teaspoon of extra virgin olive oil, **Or**

- 150 g (5.3 oz.) lean- cut meat (see 'food-source' guide for allowed selection) or turkey breast and 200 g (7 oz.) of potatoes or sweet potatoes and a small salad and a tablespoon of extra virgin olive oil on top, Or

- 200 g (7 oz.) white fish (see 'food-source' guide for selection) and a 3 to 4 pieces of fruit, **Or**

- 150 g (5.3 oz.) wild salmon and 1 cup of cooked brown rice and a small salad and teaspoon extra virgin olive oil

Meal 4

- 2 level tablespoons of natural peanut butter and 8 large rice cakes, **Or**

- 200 g (7 oz.) of white fish (refer to food sources guide for selection) and 200 g (7 oz.) potatoes or sweet potatoes, **Or**

- 2 cups of low-fat cottage cheese and 8 large rice cakes and a whole egg, **Or**

- 200 g (7 oz.) of white fish (refer to food sources guide for selection) and 1.5 cups of cooked brown rice

Meal 5

- 150 g (5.3 oz.) skinless chicken or turkey breast and 1.5 cups of cooked brown rice and a small salad and a teaspoon of extra virgin olive oil as dressing, **Or**

- 2 scoops of protein powder and 3 to 4 pieces of fruit (berries - either frozen or fresh are a great choice and 1 cup would serve as 1 to 2 pieces of fruit,) **Or**

- 150 g (5.3 oz.) of white fish (refer to 'food-sources' guide for selection) with 200 g (7 oz.) of potatoes or sweet potatoes and a small salad and a tablespoon of extra virgin olive oil as dressing

Meal 6

- 2 cups (~500 ml/g) of egg-whites and 75 g of dry cream-of-wheat, **Or**

- 2 cups of low-fat cottage cheese and 1 cup of oats, **Or**

- 2 cups (~500 ml/g) of egg-whites and 3 to 4 pieces of fruit, **Or**

- 2 tablespoons of natural peanut butter and 8 large rice cakes

Once per week sub in 150 g (7 oz.) of lean-cut steak as a protein source in place of any of the protein sources for meal 5. Keep the rest of the meal the same.

Once per week sub in 150 g (7 oz.) of wild salmon as a protein source in place of any of the protein sources for meal 5. Keep the rest of the meal the same.

~3,300 **CALORIE** MEAL PLAN

Meal 1

- 1 whole egg, 2 cups of egg-whites (~500 ml), 75 g of dry cream-of-wheat, **Or**

- 3 whole eggs, 5 egg-whites and 75 g of dry cream of wheat, **Or**

- 2 tablespoons of natural peanut butter and 1 cup of oats

Meal 2

- 30 g (0.7 oz.) of nuts (about what fits in the small palm of your hand) and 10 large rice cakes, **Or**

- 1 can of tuna packed in water and 1.5 cups of cooked long-grain brown rice and a small salad with a 1 tablespoon of extra virgin olive oil on top, **Or**

- 1 to 2 scoops of protein powder and 10 large rice cakes (preferably the first or second option)

Meal 3

- 200 g (7 oz.) shrimp drained, 1.5 cups of cooked brown rice and a small salad and a tablespoon of extra virgin olive oil, **Or**

- 200 g (7 oz.) lean-cut meat (see 'food-source' guide for allowed selection) or turkey breast and 200 g (7 oz.) of potatoes or sweet potatoes and a small salad and a tablespoon of extra virgin olive oil on top, Or

- 200 g (7 oz.) white fish (see 'food-source' guide for selection) and a 3 to 4 pieces of fruit and teaspoon of olive oil, **Or**

- 150 g (5.3 oz.) wild salmon and 1.5 cups of cooked brown rice and a small salad and teaspoon extra virgin olive oil

Meal 4

- 2 level tablespoons of natural peanut butter and 10 large plain rice cakes, **Or**

- 200 g (7 oz.) of white fish (refer to food sources guide for selection) and 250 g (8.8 oz.) potatoes or sweet potatoes, **Or**

- 1 whole egg and 2 cups of low-fat cottage cheese and 10 large rice cakes, **Or**

- 200 g (7 oz.) of white fish (refer to food sources guide for selection) and 1.5 cups of cooked brown rice

Meal 5

- 150 g (5.3 oz.) skinless chicken or turkey breast and 1.5 cups of cooked brown rice and a small salad and a teaspoon of extra virgin olive oil as dressing, **Or**

- 2 scoops of protein powder and 3 to 4 pieces of fruit (berries - either frozen or fresh are a great choice and 1 cup would serve as 1 to 2 pieces of fruit,) **Or**

- 150 g (5.3 oz.) of white fish (refer to 'food-sources' guide for selection) with 200 g (7 oz.) of potatoes or sweet potatoes and a small salad and a tablespoon of extra virgin olive oil as dressing

Meal 6

- 2 cups (~500 ml/g) of egg-whites and 75 g of dry cream-of-wheat and 1 teaspoon of natural peanut butter, **Or**

- One whole egg and 2 cups of low-fat cottage cheese and 1 cup of oats, **Or**

- 2 cups (~500 ml/g) of egg-whites and 3 to 4 pieces of fruit, **Or**

- 2 tablespoons of natural peanut butter and 10 large plain rice cakes

Once per week sub in 150 g (7 oz.) of lean-cut steak as a protein source in place of any of the protein sources for meal 5. Keep the rest of the meal the same.

Once per week sub in 150 g (7 oz.) of wild salmon as a protein source in place of any of the protein sources for meal 5. Keep the rest of the meal the same.

~3,600 **CALORIE** MEAL PLAN

Meal 1

- Two level tablespoons of natural peanut butter and 1 & 1/3 cups of dry oats, **Or**

- 3 whole eggs, 6 egg-whites and ½ of a cup of dry cream of wheat, **Or**

- Two whole eggs, 2 cups of egg-whites (~500 ml), 75 g of dry cream-of-wheat

Meal 2

- 2 scoops of protein powder and 10 large rice cakes (preferably the second or third option,) **Or**

- 30 g (1 oz.) of nuts (about what fits in the small palm of your hand) and 12 large plain rice cakes, **Or**

- 1 can of tuna packed in water and 1.5 cups of cooked long-grain brown rice and a small salad with a 1 tablespoon of extra virgin olive oil on top

Meal 3

- 200 g (7 oz.) shrimp drained, 2 cups of cooked brown rice & a small salad & a teaspoon of extra virgin olive oil, **Or**

- 200 g (7 oz.) lean-cut meat (see 'food-source' guide for allowed selection) or turkey breast and 250 g (8.8 oz.) of potatoes or sweet potatoes and a small salad and a tablespoon of extra virgin olive oil on top, Or

- 200 g (7 oz.) white fish (see 'food-source' guide for selection) and 4 pieces of fruit and tablespoon of olive oil, **Or**

- 150 g (5.3 oz.) wild salmon and 2 cups of cooked brown rice and a small salad

Meal 4

- 2 level tablespoons of natural peanut butter and 12 large plain rice cakes, **Or**

- 200 g (7 oz.) of white fish (refer to food sources guide for selection) and 250 g (8.8 oz.) potatoes or sweet potatoes and a <u>tea</u>spoon of extra virgin olive oil, **Or**

- 1 whole egg and 2 cups of low-fat cottage cheese and 11 large rice cakes, **Or**

- 200 g (7 oz.) of white fish (refer to food sources guide for selection) and 2 cups of cooked brown rice

Meal 5

- 150 g (5.3 oz.) skinless chicken or turkey breast and 1.5 cups of cooked brown rice and a small salad and a tablespoon of extra virgin olive oil as dressing, **Or**

- 2 scoops of protein powder and 4 pieces of fruit (berries - either frozen or fresh are a great choice and 1 cup would serve as 1 to 2 pieces of fruit,) **Or**

- 150 g (5.3 oz.) of white fish (refer to 'food-sources' guide for selection) with 250 g (8.8 oz.) of potatoes or sweet potatoes and a small salad and a tablespoon of extra virgin olive oil as dressing

Meal 6

- 2 cups (~500 ml/g) of egg-whites and 75 g of dry cream-of-wheat and 1 tablespoon of natural peanut butter, **Or**

- Two whole eggs and 2 cups of low-fat cottage cheese and 1 cup of oats, **Or**

- One whole egg and 2 cups (~500 ml/g) of egg-whites and 4 pieces of fruit, **Or**

- 2 tablespoons of natural peanut butter and 12 large plain rice cakes

Once per week sub in 150 g (7 oz.) of lean-cut steak as a protein source in place of any of the protein sources for meal 5. Keep the rest of the meal the same.

Once per week sub in 150 g (7 oz.) of wild salmon as a protein source in place of any of the protein sources for meal 5. Keep the rest of the meal the same.

~3,900 **CALORIE**
MEAL PLAN

Meal 1

- One whole egg and two level tablespoons of natural peanut butter and 1 & 1/3 cups of dry oats, **Or**

- 3 whole eggs and 1 cup of egg-whites and ½ of a cup of dry cream of wheat, **Or**

- Two whole eggs, 2 cups of egg-whites (~500 ml), 75 g of dry cream-of-wheat

Meal 2

- 2 scoops of protein powder and 12 large rice cakes (preferably the second or third option,) **Or**

- 1 can of tuna packed in water and 2 cups of cooked long-grain brown rice and a small salad with a 1 tablespoon of extra virgin olive oil on top, **Or**

- 35 g (1.2 oz.) of nuts (about what fits in the small palm of your hand) and 12 large plain rice cakes

Meal 3

- 200 g (7 oz.) shrimp drained, 2 cups of cooked brown rice & a small salad & a teaspoon of extra virgin olive oil, **Or**

- 200 g (7 oz.) lean- cut meat (see 'food-source' guide for allowed selection) or turkey breast and 250 g (8.8 oz.) of potatoes or sweet potatoes and a small salad and a tablespoon of extra virgin olive oil on top, Or

- 200 g (7 oz.) white fish (see 'food-source' guide for selection) and 4 pieces of fruit and tablespoon of olive oil, **Or**

- 150 g (5.3 oz.) wild salmon and 2 cups of cooked brown rice and a small salad and a teaspoon of olive oil

Meal 4

- 3 tablespoons of natural peanut butter and 10 large plain rice cakes, **Or**

- 200 g (7 oz.) of white fish (refer to food sources guide for selection) and 250 g (8.8 oz.) potatoes or sweet potatoes and 1 to 2 tablespoons of extra virgin olive oil, **Or**

- 1 whole egg and 2 cups of low-fat cottage cheese and 12 large rice cakes, **Or**

- 200 g (7 oz.) of white fish (refer to food sources guide for selection) and 2 cups of cooked brown rice

Meal 5

- 200 g (7 oz.) skinless chicken or turkey breast and 1.5 cups of cooked brown rice and a small salad and a tablespoon of extra virgin olive oil as dressing, **Or**

- 2 scoops of protein powder and 4 to 5 pieces of fruit (berries - either frozen or fresh are a great choice, and 1 cup would serve as 1 to 2 pieces of fruit) and a tablespoon of natural peanut butter, **Or**

- 200 g (7 oz.) of white fish (refer to 'food-sources' guide for selection) with 250 g (8.8 oz.) of potatoes or sweet potatoes and a small salad and a tablespoon of extra virgin olive oil as dressing

Meal 6

- 2 rounded tablespoons of natural peanut butter and 12 large plain rice cakes, **Or**

- 1 whole egg and 2 cups of low-fat cottage cheese and 1 cup of dry oats, 1 tablespoon peanut butter, **Or**

- 2 whole eggs and 2 cups (~500 ml/g) of egg-whites and 5 pieces of fruit, **Or**

- 2 cups (~500 ml/g) of egg-whites and 75 g of dry cream-of-wheat and 1 tablespoon of peanut butter

Once per week sub in 150 g (7 oz.) of lean-cut steak as a protein source in place of any of the protein sources for meal 5. Keep the rest of the meal the same.

Once per week sub in 150 g (7 oz.) of wild salmon as a protein source in place of any of the protein sources for meal 5. Keep the rest of the meal the same.

~4,200 **CALORIE** MEAL PLAN

Meal 1

- Two whole eggs, 2 cups of egg-whites (~500 ml), ½ of a cup of dry cream-of-wheat, **Or**

- 3 whole eggs, 1 cup of egg-whites, ½ a cup of dry cream of wheat and a teaspoon of natural peanut butter, **Or**

- Three level tablespoons of natural peanut butter and 1 & 1/3 cups of dry oats

Meal 2

- 1 can of tuna packed in water and 2 cups of cooked long-grain brown rice and a small salad with a 1 to 2 tablespoons of extra virgin olive oil on top, **Or**

- 2.5 scoops of protein powder and 12 large rice cakes (preferably the second or third option,) **Or**

- 40 g (1.5 oz.) of nuts and 12 large plain rice cakes

Meal 3

- 200 g (7 oz.) white fish (see 'food-source' guide for selection), 4 pieces of fruit and 1 to 2 tablespoons of olive oil, **Or**

- 200 g (7 oz.) lean- cut meat (see 'food-source' guide for allowed selection) or turkey breast and 250 g (8.8 oz.) of potatoes or sweet potatoes and a small salad and 1 to 2 tablespoons of extra virgin olive oil on top, Or

- 200 g (7 oz.) shrimp drained, 2 cups of cooked brown rice & a small salad and a tablespoon of extra virgin olive oil, **Or**

- 200 g (7 oz.) wild salmon and 2 cups of cooked brown rice and a small salad and a teaspoon of olive oil

Meal 4

- Two whole eggs and 2 cups of low-fat cottage cheese and 12 large rice cakes, **Or**

- 200 g (7 oz.) of white fish (refer to food sources guide for selection) and 300 g (10.5 oz.) potatoes or sweet potatoes and 1 to 2 tablespoons of extra virgin olive oil, **Or**

- 3 tablespoons of natural peanut butter and 12 large plain rice cakes, **Or**

- 200 g (7oz.) of white fish (refer to food sources guide for selection), 2 cups of cooked brown rice, 1 tablespoon Olive oil

Meal 5

- 200 g (7 oz.) skinless chicken or turkey breast and 1.5 cups of cooked brown rice and a small salad and 1 to 2 tablespoons of extra virgin olive oil as dressing, **Or**

- 2 scoops of protein powder and 4 to 5 pieces of fruit (berries - either frozen or fresh are a great choice and 1 cup would serve as 1 to 2 pieces of fruit) and 2 tablespoons of natural peanut butter, **Or**

- 200 g (7 oz.) of white fish (refer to 'food-sources' guide for selection) with 300 g (10.5 oz.) of potatoes or sweet potatoes and a small salad and a tablespoon of extra virgin olive oil as dressing

Meal 6

- 1 whole egg and 2 cups (~500 ml/g) of egg-whites and 5 pieces of fruit, 1 tablespoon peanut butter, **Or**

- 2 cups of low-fat cottage cheese and 1 cup of dry oats, 2 tablespoons peanut butter, **Or**

- 3 tablespoons of natural peanut butter and 12 large plain rice cakes, **Or**

- 2 cups (~500 ml/g) of egg-whites and 75 g of dry cooked cream-of-wheat and 2 tablespoons of peanut butter

Once per week sub in 150 g (7 oz.) of lean-cut steak as a protein source in place of any of the protein sources for meal 5. Keep the rest of the meals the same.

Once per week sub in 150 g (7 oz.) of wild salmon as a protein source in place of any of the protein sources for meal 5. Keep the rest of the meal the same.

BONUSES

Formatted Workouts

Again, the Kindle file format is not ideal for a workout program. To get the free, formatted, and printable version of all 80 workouts in The Hardgainer Solution, please visit:

scottabelfitness.com/hgsworkouts/

Exercise Library

I mentioned it at the beginning of the list of workouts, but if you need to see a demonstration of any video, go to my website to browse **my video exercise library** at:

scottabelfitness.com/library/

Even if you're familiar with every exercise, I think you'll find it useful to see my explanations of really important movements like the Squat and the Bench Press.

If you have been paying attention, you will notice that I emphasize form and technique as well as *execution* and *application.*

Doing a squat in order to lift the most weight you can, even with "proper form," is actually totally different than squatting to build huge legs. Same goes for Bench Press. That is what a lot of my videos get into.

"What Program Should I Do Next?"

After doing the workouts in Hardgainer Solution, any of my programs would be a good pick, as you will be better equipped to handle volume and hit your muscles properly.

You can try a traditional five or six-day split, and you should find that you are better able to target individual muscles, and to recover workout to workout and within a single workout. But then again you also might really enjoy the flexibility of whole body training, and you could continue on in that vein.

Learn More

To learn more about diet, training, and physique transformation, or to get announcements about future books, please visit my website and subscribe to my email list: **https://scottabelfitness.com/**. I send out free articles on nutrition and working out, as well as case studies, client updates, and more.

If you liked this book, and want to see more, please take a moment to write a review on Amazon and let me know!

Thank you for purchasing and taking the time to read this book. I appreciate it, and I hope you get a lot out of it.

DISCLAIMER AND/OR LEGAL NOTICES:

Every effort has been made to accurately represent this book and it's potential. Results vary with every individual, and your results may or may not be different from those depicted. No promises, guarantees or warranties, whether stated or implied, have been made that you will produce any specific result from this book. Your efforts are individual and unique, and may vary from those shown. Your success depends on your efforts, background and motivation.

The material in this publication is provided for educational and informational purposes only and is not intended as medical advice. The information contained in this book should not be used to diagnose or treat any illness, metabolic disorder, disease or health problem. Always consult your physician or health care provider before beginning any nutrition or exercise program. Use of the programs, advice, and information contained in this book is at the sole choice and risk of the reader.

40569114R00146

Made in the USA
Middletown, DE
16 February 2017